Veterinary Entomology and Acarology

NIPA® GENX ELECTRONIC RESOURCES & SOLUTIONS P. LTD.
New Delhi-110 034

About the Authors

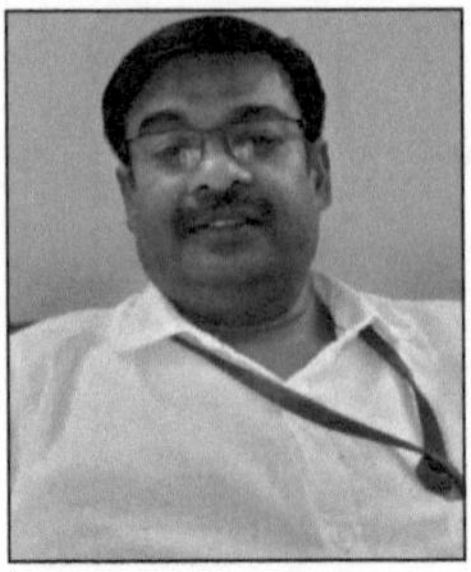

Dr. Amit Singh, presently, is serving as a Professor & Head in Department of Veterinary Parasitology, Acharya Narendra Deva University of Agriculture & Technology, Kumarganj, Ayodhya, Uttar Pradesh. He has more than 24 years of teaching, research and extension experience. Dr. Singh did his Bachelor of Veterinary Science and Animal Husbandry (B.V.Sc. & A.H.) degree in 1997 followed by MVSc in Veterinary Parasitology in 2000 from Chaudhary Charan Singh Haryana Agriculture University, Hisar, Haryana. Later as an in-service candidate, he completed his Ph.D. in Veterinary Parasitology from DUVASU, Mathura. Before joining ANDUAT, Dr. Singh also worked as Research Associate at CCS, HAU, Hisar under NATP project where he extensively worked on the prevalence and immunodiagnosis of Schistosomosis in domestic animals. At ANDUAT, he is credited with establishment of Molecular lab in Department of Veterinary Parasitology with the help of RKVY project. Currently, he is Principal Investigator of project granted by UP Council of Agriculture Research on ticks management in Eastern Uttar Pradesh. He has guided six MVSc and two Ph.D students and till date published three books, 54 research articles in reputed national and international Journals and numerous technical/popular articles. He has organized several training programmes and workshops for the Veterinary Officers, Livestock Extension Officers, paravets and farmers of Uttar Pradesh. Dr. Singh is a member of Indian Association for the Advancement of Veterinary Parasitology (IAAVP), Society of Immunology and Immunopathology and UP Veterinary Council. He has also acted as a reviewer of several research articles of various reputed journals besides being an expert member for the selection of Assistant Professor in several organizations.

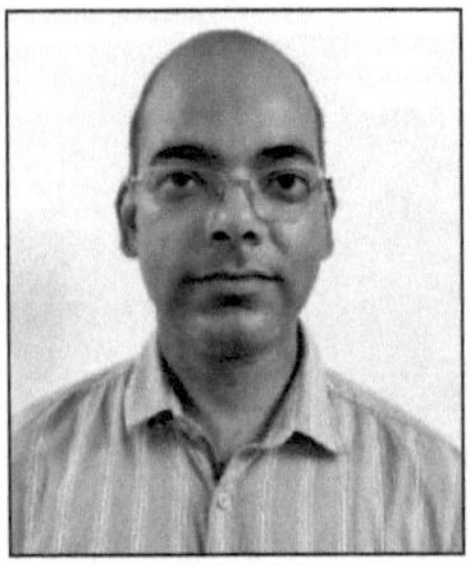

Dr. Amit Kumar Jaiswal hails from the Bareilly district of Uttar Pradesh, where he completed his early education. He earned his Bachelor of Veterinary Science and Animal Husbandry (B.V.Sc. & A.H.) degree in 2006 from Chandra Shekhar Azad University of Agriculture & Technology, Kanpur, Uttar Pradesh. Dr. Jaiswal secured the prestigious ICAR-Junior Research Fellowship (JRF) for his Master's program and subsequently completed his M.V.Sc. in Veterinary Parasitology from G.B. Pant University of Agriculture & Technology, Pantnagar, Uttarakhand in 2009. He further advanced his academic credentials by obtaining an in-service Ph.D. in Veterinary Parasitology in 2018. Dr. Jaiswal's professional journey commenced as a Veterinary Officer with the U.P. Government, a role he served from September 2008 to April 2010. He then transitioned to academia, joining the Department of

Veterinary Parasitology at the College of Veterinary Science, DUVASU, Mathura as an Assistant Professor on April 28, 2010, and was subsequently elevated to the position of Associate Professor on April 28, 2023. He is a distinguished lifetime member of several eminent organizations, including the Indian Association for the Advancement of Veterinary Parasitology (IAAVP), The Indian Science Congress Association, Kolkata, and the Indian Society of Veterinary Medicine (ISVM). Dr. Jaiswal has actively engaged in a multitude of trainings, conferences workshops, and symposia. He also had the honor of being a visiting scholar at the University of Illinois at Urbana-Champaign, Illinois, USA. In recognition of his innovative contributions, Dr. Jaiswal was awarded a patent by the Patent Office Government of India, as the principal inventor for his creation, "An essential oil-based formulation for control of *Rhipicephalus microplus* tick." His prolific academic output includes six laboratory manuals, numerous popular articles, book chapters, a book, and over 50 research articles published in esteemed national and international journals.

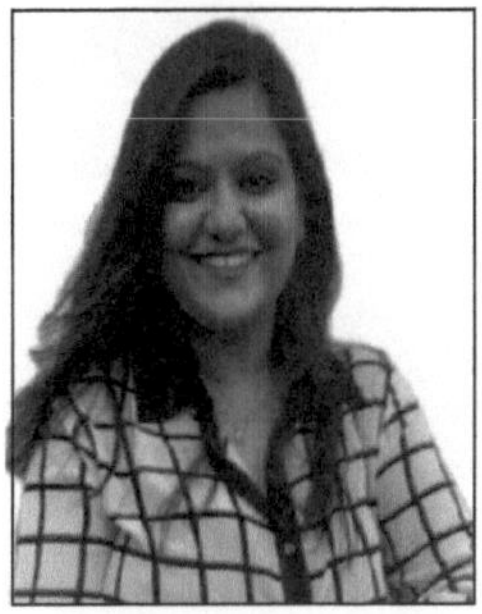

Dr. Supriya Sachan was born in the Kanpur District of Uttar Pradesh, embarked on her academic journey in veterinary sciences with a Bachelor of Veterinary Science and Animal Husbandry (B.V. Sc & A.H.) degree in 2018 from U.P. Pandit Deen Dayal Upadhyaya Pashu Chikitsa Vigyan Vishwavidyalaya Evam Go-Anusandhan Sansthan (DUVASU), Mathura, Uttar Pradesh. She further pursued her M.V. Sc in Veterinary Parasitology at Nanaji Deshmukh Veterinary Science University, Jabalpur, graduating in 2020. In 2023, Dr. attained her Ph.D. from Guru Angad Dev Veterinary and Animal Sciences University, Ludhiana, where she was awarded a university merit scholarship. That same year, she commenced her tenure as an Assistant Professor in the Department of Veterinary Parasitology at the College of Veterinary Science and Animal Husbandry, DUVASU, Mathura. Dr. is a lifetime member of the Indian Association for the Advancement of Veterinary Parasitology (IAAVP) and the Association of Animal Scientists (AAS).

Veterinary Entomology and Acarology

Amit Singh
Professor & Head
Department of Veterinary Parasitology
College of Veterinary Science and Animal Husbandry, Kumarganj
Acharya Narendra Deva University of Agriculture & Technology
Kumarganj, Ayodhya, Uttar Pradesh-224 229

Amit Kumar Jaiswal
Associate Professor
Department of Veterinary Parasitology
College of Veterinary Science and Animal Husbandry
U.P. Pandit Deen Dayal Upadhyaya Pashu Chikitsa Vigyan Vishwavidyalaya
Evam Go-Anusandhan Sansthan (DUVASU)
Mathura, Uttar Pradesh-281 001

Supriya Sachan
Assistant Professor
Department of Veterinary Parasitology
College of Veterinary Science and Animal Husbandry
U.P. Pandit Deen Dayal Upadhyaya Pashu Chikitsa Vigyan Vishwavidyalaya
Evam Go-Anusandhan Sansthan (DUVASU)
Mathura, Uttar Pradesh-281 001

NIPA® GENX ELECTRONIC RESOURCES & SOLUTIONS P. LTD.
New Delhi-110 034

NIPA® GENX ELECTRONIC
RESOURCES & SOLUTIONS P. LTD.
101,103, Vikas Surya Plaza, CU Block
L.S.C.Market, Pitam Pura, New Delhi-110 034
Ph : +91 11 4386 0225, 9717133558, 9540816132
E-mail: newindiapublishingagency@gmail.com
Website: www.niparesources.com

For customer assistance, please contact
Phone: + 91-11-27 34 17 17
Fax: + 91-11-27 34 16 16
E-Mail: feedbacks@nipabooks.com

Print ISBN: 978-93-58879-64-3

ebook ISBN: 978-93-58873-60-3

Composed and Designed by NIPA®.

Acknowledgements

At the very outset with folded hands, we bow our head with reverence to the "ALMIGHTY GOD" and will forever be grateful to God for giving us right directions with right people in our life and helped us sail smoothly through this endeavour.

Mere words of acknowledgement will never express our heartfelt and sincerest feelings of gratitude, indebtedness and thankfulness to honourable Vice Chancellors of Acharya Narendra Deva University of Agriculture & Technology, Kumarganj, Ayodhya (U.P.) 224 229 and U.P. Pandit Deen Dayal Upadhyaya Pashu Chikitsa Vigyan Vishwavidyalaya Evam Go-Anusandhan Sansthan (DUVASU), Mathura (U.P.) 281 001 for able guidance, constant encouragement and support.

Authors owe their earnest and whole hearted thanks to the faculty members and associated staff in department of Veterinary Parasitology of both the colleges at ANDUAT, Kumarganj, Ayodhya, and DUVASU, Mathura for rendering help and moral support in bringing this book to fruition.

Authors are thankful to Ishan Garg, Khyati Srivastava, and Shivkesh, 3rd professional B.V.Sc. & A.H students of College of Veterinary Science and Animal Husbandry, DUVASU, Mathura, who created the beautiful line diagrams featured in this book. Authors also acknowledge Dr. Kale Chandrakant Dinkar M.V.Sc scholar, Department of Veterinary Parasitology, DUVASU, Mathura for his contribution to a book chapter.

Amit Singh
Amit Kumar Jaiswal
Supriya Sachan

Preface

Arthropods, comprising over 80% of Earth's living organisms and play a vital role to the animal industry. These invertebrates, many of which are ectoparasites, inhabit the bodies of hosts, causing numerous detrimental effects to both animals and humans. Their significance extends beyond their pathogenic effects, as they also function as vectors for major diseases such as Trypanosomosis, Theileriosis, and Blue Tongue in livestock, additionally they transmit various human diseases, including Lyme disease, Tularemia, and Kyasanur Forest Disease. The economic impact caused by the class Arachnida amounts to 46,199.31 million INR, underscoring that the cumulative damage inflicted by the entire phylum Arthropoda can significantly disrupt the livestock industry. Consequently, a comprehensive understanding of this phylum is essential for developing effective control and management strategies. Recognizing their importance, the Veterinary Council of India has established a specialized course, "Arthropods of Veterinary Importance," for veterinary graduates.

This book aims to elucidate the key morphological characteristics, life cycles significance, pathogenesis, control, and treatment of major arthropod parasites relevant to veterinary science. It includes detailed line diagrams highlighting essential morphological features for accurate identification. Additionally, the book addresses integrated pest management and acaricide resistance, providing readers with up-to-date strategies for managing arthropods. A dedicated chapter on common laboratory techniques in entomology and acarology will guide readers in preserving arthropod specimens for educational and research purposes. The authors have thoughtfully structured the text into bullet points where necessary, facilitating quick topic recaps.

The authors aspire for this book to be a valuable resource for undergraduate and postgraduate students, veterinary practitioners, and biologists in the teaching and learning of this subject.

Amit Singh
Amit Kumar Jaiswal
Supriya Sachan

Contents

Acknowledgements ... *vii*

Preface ... *ix*

1. Introduction to Arthropods ... 1
2. General Characters of Class Insecta ... 7
3. Classification of Class Insecta ... 13
4. Order Diptera ... 15
5. Order Coleoptera ... 63
6. Order Siphonptera ... 65
7. Order Mallophaga and Siphunculata ... 73
8. Order Hemiptera ... 85
9. Order Orthoptera and Odonata ... 89
10. Important Characters and Classification of Class Arachnida ... 91
11. Soft Ticks (Argasidae) ... 95
12. Hard Ticks (Ixodidae) ... 101
13. Mites ... 129
14. Pentastomida ... 147
15. Integrated Pest Management (IPM) ... 149
16. Acaricide Resistance ... 159
17. Common Laboratory Techniques in Entomology and Acarology ... 167

Annexures 175

Annexure 1: Preparation of Common Laboratory Reagents and Solutions For Arthropods 175

Annexure 2: List of Arthropods of Veterinary Importance in Tabular form 176

Annexure 3: Important Vector-Borne Diseases of Canine 184

Annexure 4: Important Vector-Borne Diseases of Cattle 185

Index *187*

1

Introduction to Arthropods

Entomology is the science, which deals with study of arthropods which parasitize or affect the domesticated animals. Since these arthropods can cause damage or injury to their host by several ways, thorough understanding of the subject is very essential. Most of these arthropods are ectoparasites living on the body of the host or at the most in subcutaneous tissues while very few are endoparasites, living inside the body of the host. Similarly, most of the arthropods are temporary parasites, while very few like lice and mites are permanent parasites. Arthropods comprise of more than 80% of living creatures on earth.

Harmful Effects Caused by Arthropods to the Body of the Host

1. **Injury to the skin**: Most of the arthropods have biting tendency and cause injury to the skin by bites. As a result, micro-wounds are produced on the body which may later on be infected with bacteria leading to localised or generalised pyoderma condition or pyodermatic patches. Similarly, such wounds are predisposed to attack of blow flies which cause a condition called as "Blow fly myiasis." Animals in order to escape the attack of flies try to run all around leading to phenomenon known as **"Entomophobia"**.
2. **Blood sucking Habits:** Most of the arthropods have blood sucking tendency like mosquitoes and ticks which may lead to anaemia.
3. **Release toxins:** Few of the arthropods release poisonous substances while biting. They inject certain poisons and toxins in the body of host. Eg. Some species of ticks release toxins causing paralysis in host known as tick paralysis.
4. **Transmission of diseases:** Arthropods have ability to transmit various bacterial, viral, protozoal, helminthic and mycotic pathogens. While sucking blood, they collect infective stages of the organism and while biting to the other host, they transmit the pathogens.

5. **Development of disease condtion**: Some arthropods cause different disease condition in the body of host like Mange and Myiasis.

Phylum Arthropoda

Phylum-Arthropoda -derived from two Greek words, “Arthos” means joints and “Podos” means legs so, the arthropods can be defined as invertebrates having joint appendages. E.g. Insects, Ticks and Mites. In terms of Veterinary importance, the arthropods can be divided into two major classes viz. Insecta and Arachnida

The branch of science which deals with the study of Insects is known as **“Entomology”** while the branch which deals with the study of arachnids (Ticks and Mites) is known as **“Acarology”.**

These arthopods are said to be descended down from the ancestors who also give origin to Annelid worms. e.g. Earthworm.

Different Characters of Phylum Arthropoda

1. They have jointed appendages or legs. The appendages of most primitive arthropods are **biramous**: having unbranched basal piece, the protopodite which branched into inner endopodite and outer exopodite.
2. Body of arthropods is **metamerically segmented** i.e. adjacent segments are morphologically identical and each segment usually has got one pair of appendages.
3. Body of arthropods is covered by a chitinous layer called as **Exoskeleton**. This layer is secreted by a chitinous glands which are located just below the exoskeleton. This chitinous layer also passes inside the mouth and cover anterior part of alimentary canal. This anterior part of alimentary canal which is lined by exoskeleton is known as **Stomodaeum**. Similarly, at posterior part, there is an invagination of exoskeleton from anus which is known as **Proctodaeum**.

   Each segment is formed by fusion of chitinous plates called as **Sclerites**. Sclerite present on dorsal aspect of the body is known as **“Tergum”** and on ventral aspect is known as **“Sternum”** and two lateral sclerites are known as **Pleurons**. As the arthropod grows in size, periodically the exoskleton is casted off and new exoskeleton of bigger size is formed and this process is known as **“Ecdysis”**. On contrary, the endoskeleton is chitinous rod which emerges out from the exoskeleton and is attached to muscular layer of the arthropod body. During the process of ecdysis along with exoskeleton, the endoskeleton is also casted off and every time new exo and endoskleton is formed i.e. Series of Ecdysis.

4. **Tagma formation or tagmosis:** Body of arthropods is metamerically segmented. In some of arthropods, i.e. highly evolved species, segments are fused to form different body regions and these body regions are called "Tagmas." e.g. In Insects, segments are fused to form 3 Tagmas i.e. Head, Thorax and Abdomen. When the segments are fused, respective appendages also modifiy into some different structures to perform different functions e.g. In Insects, the appendages of segments which are fused to form head are modified into eyes, antenna and mouth parts. In the thorax region, appendages remain for locomotion. Appendages of abdominal segments are usually lost in terrestrial insects i.e. land insects while in "aquatic insects" abdominal appendages are retained for locomotion in water.
5. **Body cavity:** In arthropods body cavity is present
6. **Different Systems of Arthropods**

A. **Digestive system:** It consist of alimentary canal which is divided into 3 parts, anterior part is **Stomodaeum** (anterior gut) posterior part is **Proctodaeum** (posterior gut) and the middle portion is known as **Mesenteron** (mid gut). Stomodaeum includes mouth, pharynx, oesophagus (crop) and proventriculus. The anterior gut or stomodaeum is concerned primarily with the ingestion and storage of food. Between the anterior gut and the mid gut, a valve is present, called the proventriculus or gizzard. **Digestion and absorption of the nutrients takes place in mesenteron since exoskleton is not present.** The cellular lining of mesentron also secretes enzymes for digestion. The hindgut ends in the rectum, having functions of absorption of water and the formation of faeces. There is a gap between alimentary canal and outer surface in form of body cavity. In arthropods, this body cavity is filled with blood coloured fluid and the cavity is called **haemocoel.**

B. **Respiratory system**: There are different types of respiratory organs depending upon the habitat of arthropods. In all aquatic arthropods, gills are present for respiration. The terrestrial arthropods have tracheal tubes. These tracheal tubes are elastic tubes covered with chitinous layer and they branch and rebranch in the body of arthropods. External opening of tracheal system is known as **Stigmata/spiracles.** Oxygen enters through the respiratory openings and passes down the trachea, usually by diffusion and a concentration gradient. Some arthropods breathe through **external surface (skin). e.g. Mites**. Some arthropods have **lung books (spider)** and **gill books (crabs).**

C. **Excretory system:** Consist of a set of tubules called as **Malpighian tubules**. Malpighian are blind at one end while other end opens in anterior part of proctodeum. Nitrogenous wastes from body of arthropods are excreted out from the haemolymph by these malpighian tubules. In class Arachnida, besides malphigian tubules, there is additional excretory organ called coxal glands which opens in the coxae of legs. **This coxal glands is true nephridia similar to crustaceans.**

D. **Nervous system**: Arthropods show a complex nervous system associated with the well-developed sense organs (eyes and antennae). The central nervous system consists of central cerebral ganglion which is located on the dorsal side of oesophagus and from this central cerebral part gives rise into two branches which surrounds the oesophagus. This loop or ring is known as **Circum-Oesophagal Commissures**. From the ventral aspect of oesophagus, this loop is continued as double nerve cord towards the posterior side of body and on each segment ganglion is present. The associated sense organs are eyes, antenna (olfactory in function) and setae. Setae are sensory hair present on the body of arthropods.

E. **Circulatory system:** It consists of a heart, aorta and haemocoele. Analogous to the blood in the vertebrates, there is fliud called **haemolymph** that circulates in the arthropods. Heart is present on dorsal aspect of arthropod body and it is tube like. It is divided into several compartments by the presence of valves, which allows haemocoele to flow only in forward direction towards the head. On either side of each compartment, there is opening known as **Ostia,** through which the haemolymph enters in heart and then is propelled through valves towards anterior side. At anterior side of heart, there is small tube called as aorta which carries the fluid to the head region and from there it enters into the haemocoel. The haemolymph is responsible for transportation of hormones, nutrients and wastes. The haemolymph lacks respiratory pigment such as haemoglobin and thus, not involved in exchange of oxygen.

F. **Reproductive system:** Arthropods are unisexual.

Male reproductive system: There are two testes, each lead to "vas deferens". At distal end of vas deferens, there is dilatation called **"Seminal Vesicles."** These two vas deferens unite to form common ejaculatory duct and terminal part is penis or **aedeagus**. The accessory sex glands produce a secretion that may help to form a packet called a spermatophore. The spermatophore encloses and protects the sperm during insemination.

Female reproductive system: The female has two ovaries each of which consists of a set of tubules. Ovary leads to oviduct which is very small and two oviducts fused to form common oviduct, which has got a dilated portion at distal end which is known as **receptaculum seminalis**. The tactile portion of oviduct is known as **ovipositor** through which eggs are laid. In most of cases, the sperms are delivered directly to the female during copulation. Sperms are usually stored in spermathecae in female. After ovulation the egg passes down the oviduct and is fertilised by sperm released from the spermathecae.

Moulting in arthropods

Arthropods shed their exoskeleton periodically which is called as **moulting or ecdysis**. The epidermis of arthropods develop new cuticle or exoskeleton before shedding of previous one. The forms of arthropods between two moultings are called as **stages or stadia** while morphologically distinct life cycle stages are called **instars**.

Phylum: Arthropoda

Phylum arthropoda comprises of different classes: -

Class: Crustacae

Class: Myriapoda

Class: Insecta

Class: Arachnida

Class: Crustacae

Most of the crustacean arthropods are aquatic and breathe through gills. The head comprises of two pairs of antennae and legs are present on thorax as well as on abdomen e.g: Crabs, cray fish, cyclops and lobster. Important from veterinary fields are crabs, crayfish which act as intermediate host for *Paragonimus westermanii* (lung fluke) while cyclops act as an intermediate host for *Diphylobothrium latum* (tapeworm), *Dracanculus* spp, *Gnathosoma* spp. (roundworms).

Class: Myriapoda

They look like earthworms but body is segmented. There is a head and fused thorax – abdomen. On thorax and abdominal segments, there may be one or two pair of appendages. Class myriapoda is divided into two sub classes:

Sub class: Diplopoda **(Millipedes)**

Sub class: Chilopoda **(Centipedes)**

In diplopoda, on each thoracic and abdomen segments, two pairs of legs. In chilopoda, there is one pair of legs. Some of these are very poisonous.

Class: Insecta

Body is divided into three tagmas; head, thorax and abdomen. On head- antennae, eyes and mouth parts are present. On thorax- three pair of legs and two pair of wings. On abdominal segments, most of insects have no appendages. E.g. flies, fleas, lice, bugs, beetles, cockroaches.

Class: Arachnida

Body is divided into cephalothorax and abdomen. Four pairs of legs are present on thorax. E.g. spider, scorpion, ticks and mites.

Class: Pentastomida: The Tongue worm or *Linguatula serrata* comes under this class.

Brief History

<table>
<tr><td>Herbert Osborn</td><td>Father of Veterinary Entomology</td></tr>
<tr><td>G.H.F. Nuttal</td><td>Founder of Medical Entomology</td></tr>
<tr><td>Patrick Manson, 1878</td><td>Mosquito Culex was vector of filarial worm Wuchereria bancrofti in human</td></tr>
<tr><td>Smith & Kilborne,1893</td><td>Tick Boophilus annulatus is the causal agent of texas fever in cattle. It carries Babesia bigemina.</td></tr>
<tr><td>Bruce, 1895</td><td>Pathogen of Nagana disease is Glossina fly</td></tr>
<tr><td>Ronald Ross, 1897</td><td>Malaria zygote in mosquitoes</td></tr>
<tr><td>Grassi, 1899</td><td>Human malaria parasite transmitted by Anopheles</td></tr>
<tr><td colspan="2">Initially, in 1880, Carlos Finlay revealed that mosquitoes transmit yellow fever which later in 1900 was proved by United State Yellow Fever Commission that it is transmitted by mosquito Aedes aegypti.</td></tr>
</table>

2

General Characters of Class Insecta

Class: Insecta

It is the biggest class in animal kingdom. About 70% of species of animals are included in class insecta.

General Morphological Characters

1. All the character of arthropoda are also present in this class.
2. Body is divided into three tagmas i.e. head, thorax and abdomen.

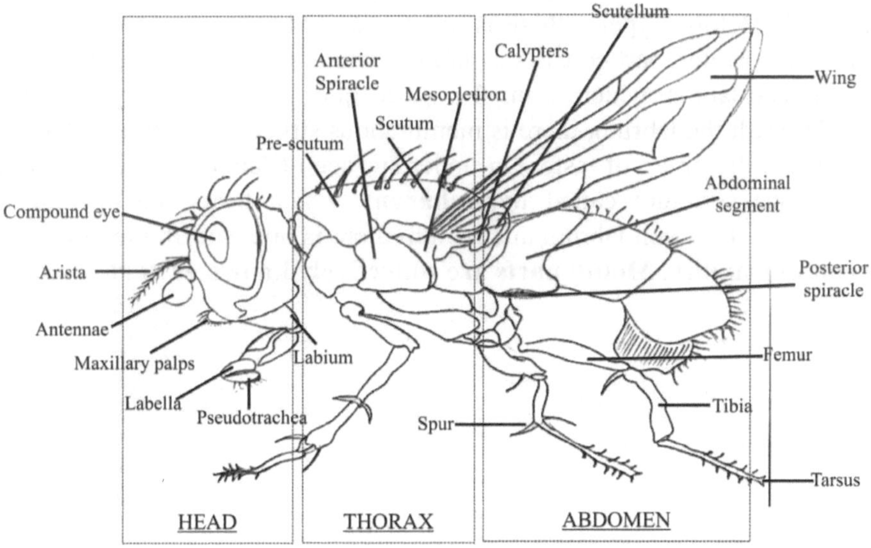

Figure 2.1. General morphological characters of insects

Normally body of arthropods consists of twenty segments. Head region is formed by the fusion of 1st six segments. Thorax is formed by next three segments and abdomen formed by last 11 segments.

Modification of six pair of appendages of head: 1st pair of appendages is modified into eyes. 2nd pair is modified into antennae. 3rd pair is lost. 4th pair of appendages is modified into mandible. 5th pair modified into first maxillae and 6th pair modified into 2nd maxillae means **mouth part is nothing but modification of 4th, 5th and 6th pair of appendages**. On abdomen, appendages or legs are lost.

Morphology of head region of insects

Highest point of head known as "**Vertex**". Anterior portion sloping in forward direction known as "**Frons**". Posterior portion sloping towards thorax is "**Occiput**". On the medial aspect of head, there is a pair of compound eyes. Each compound eye is made of number of lenses called as "**facet**". Compound eyes may meet one another in mid line (**holoptic**) or are wide apart (**dichoptic**). Just medial to compound eyes, there is a pair of non-functioning simple eyes known as "**ocellus.**" Just in front of these two eyes on either side, there is a pair of antennae. Antennae are made up of three parts, base, pedicle and filaments. Pedicle is non segment basal piece. On these antennae, hair may be present. At the base of each antenna, there is olfactory pin. Lateral part of head is known as "**Gena**". Just below the frons, there is a chitinous plate known as "**Clypeus**". Below clypeus, there is mouth part. Mouth parts are located on ventral side. Mouth part consists of labrum which forms the upper boundary of mouth and labium which forms the lower lip or lower boundary of mouth. On underneath the labrum, there is membranous structure called **epipharynx** which bears the organ of taste. On upper surface of labium, there is another membranous structure called **hypopharynx** which bears the opening of salivary duct. Between labrum and labium there is one pair of mandibles and one pair of maxillae. **Mouth parts are collectively known as "Proboscis"**.

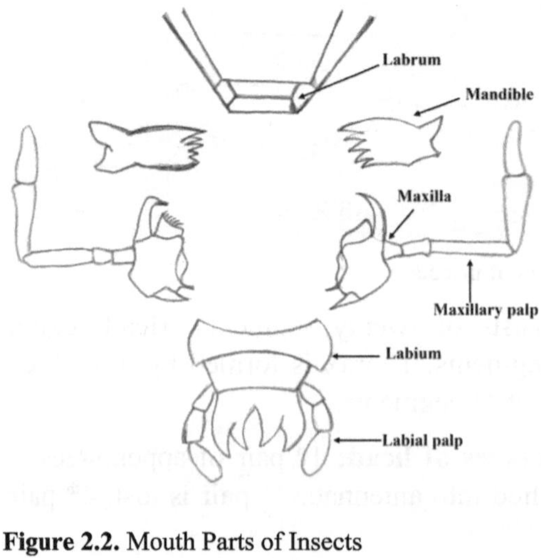

Figure 2.2. Mouth Parts of Insects

Depending upon the type of food habit of insect, there are adaptations in mouth parts:

1. Biting and chewing type of mouth parts: eg. Cockroach
2. Piercing and sucking type of mouth parts: eg. Mosquitoes
3. Cutting and sucking type of mouth parts: eg. *Stomoxys*
4. Cutting and sponging type of mouth parts: eg. *Tabanus*
5. Sponging or Lapping type of mouth parts: eg. *Musca*

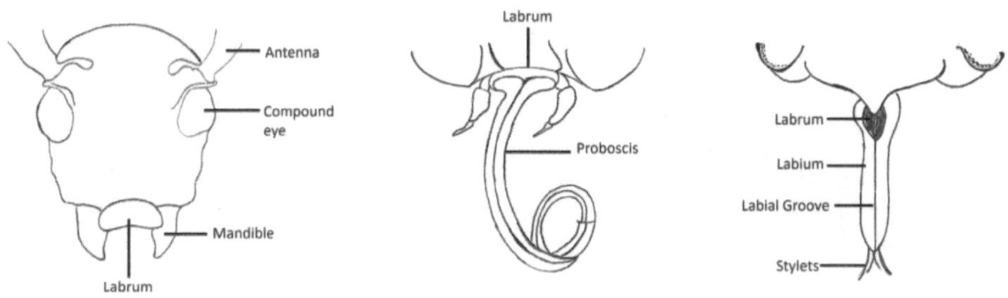

Figure 2.3. Adaptations in mouth parts

Morphology of thorax: Thorax is made up of 3 segments. First segment is known as "Prothorax.", second segment is known as "Mesothorax" and third segment is known as "Metathorax." On each thoracic segment there is a pair of legs. Two pair of wings are present, 1st pair of wings on mesothorax and 2nd pair on metathorax.

Morphology of legs: Legs comprises of basal coxa by which legs are attached to the body. It is followed by triangular structure called as "trochanter", followed by one elongated piece called as "femur" then one more elongated piece called as "tibia" and lastly "tarsii." On the tarsus, there may be presence of one or two claws. In some insects, there is a pair of soft pads in between two claws known as **"Pulvillus"** and a stiff bristle arising from pulvillus known as **"Empodium".**

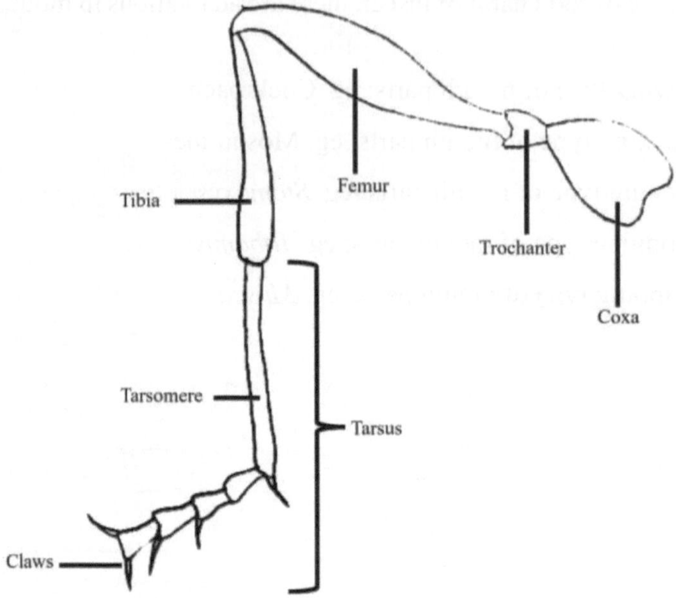

Figure 2.4. Parts of leg of insects

Morphology of wings: Each wing consists of two membranous structures which are attached to each other very firmly. Between these two membranes, tracheal tube runs and these are referred as "veins of wing" and this has got diagnostic importance as on the basis of veinous pattern, different insects are identified. Veins are also named as:

1st pair- Costa

2nd pair- Subcosta

3rd pair- Radial

4th pair- Median

5th pair- Cubital

6th pair- Anal

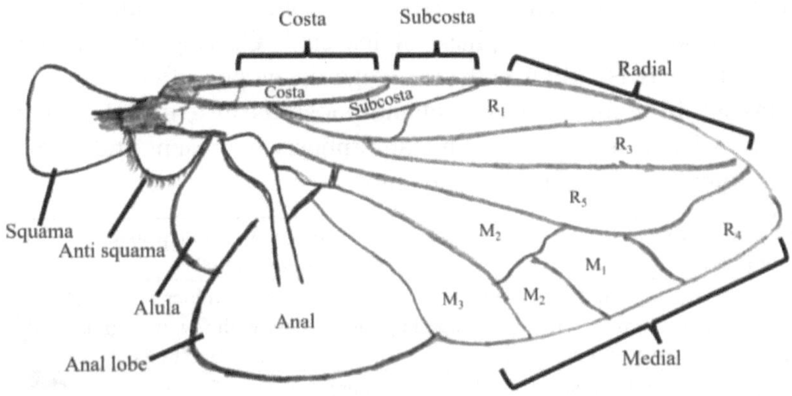

Figure 2.5. Morphology of insect wing

First four veins (1st, 2nd, 3rd and 4th) are referred as longitudinal veins while 5th and 6th as horizontal veins. Each wing has got an anterior straight margin, posterior convex margin, base and apex. Basal segment of the wing is known as "**Squamma**".

Morphology of Abdomen: It is soft and membranous and made up of eleven segment and appendages are lost. The tenth and eleventh segments are usually small and not visible externally. The eleventh segment is lost in most advanced groups of Insecta. The genital ducts open ventrally on the abdominal segment 8 or 9 and often bear external organs to assist in reproduction. The genitalia are composed of structures originated from abdominal appendages. In male insect, the basic external genitalia consist of one or two pairs of **claspers**, which hold the female during copulation. In female, there is a specialised appendicular **ovipositor**, made up of appendages on the terminal segments of the abdomen, or the tip of the abdomen may be elongated at the time of oviposition to form a simpler substitutional ovipositor.

Development of Insects

Depending upon reproductive stage, there are 4 types of insects:

i. Oviparous insects – The insects lay eggs.

ii. Larviparous insects – The insects lay larvae e.g. *Oestrus ovis.*

iii. Pupiparous insects – The insects laid larvae in advance stage of developments, immediately after deposition of larvae, they moult to next stage i.e. pupa. e.g. *Glossina fly*.

iv. Parthenogenetic – The development of insect without fertilization. eg. Bees and Wasp.

Metamorphosis: It is defined as "series of morphological changes that are taking place in post embryonic phase of insects". **Casting of exoskeleton during development is called ecdyses**. Stage developed after each ecdyses is called **instar.** In some insects, metamorphosis is absent and known as **Ametamorphosis.** In most insects, metamorphosis is present and is of two types either complete or incomplete metamorphosis.

Complete metamorphosis (Holometabolous)	**Incomplete metamorphosis (Hemimetabolous)**
There is a complete change in morphology. Larval stage does not resemble with adult stage in morphology. e.g. Butterfly and caterpillar.	Larval stage resembles with adult stage except with few morphological differences. e.g. Bed bugs.
Sudden change in morphology, so period of moult is very short.	There is a gradual change.
Resting stage is present called as pupa.	Pupal stage is absent and nymph is present.
Life cycle stages are: Eggs- larva-**pupa (Chrysalis)** -Imago -adult.	Life cycle stages are: Egg- larva- **nymph**- adult.

Types of larvae

In class insecta on basis of presence of legs the larvae can be divided into three

1) **Polypodous larva:** Legs are present on thorax as well as on abdomen. eg. Butterfly and caterpillar.
2) **Oligopodous larva:** Legs are present only on thorax. Eg. Beetles.
3) **Apodous larva:** Legs are absent. Apodous larva is also called "**Maggots**". e.g. Different flies like *Musca* and *Stomoxys*.

Types of pupa

Three types of pupa are noticed in class Insecta

1) **Free or Exarate pupa:** Outer covering of pupa is transparent and wings and legs of insects can be seen externally. Wings and legs are free from the body. e.g. Beetles.
2) **Obtectate pupa:** Outer covering is transparent but legs and wings are not free. They are attached to body by moulting fluid.e.g. Mosquitoes.
3) **Coaractate pupa:** Outer wall is very thick so not transparent and here outer wall is known as "**Puparium".** In these insects, exoskeleton of last larval stage is retained on the pupa e.g. Flies.

3

Classification of Class Insecta

Classification of Class Insecta

Subclass

Apterygota	Pterygota
Wings are absent.	Wings are present or may be wingless.
Metamorphosis is absent.	Metamorphosis is present.
One or more pair of abdominal appendages is present other than genitalia and cerci.	No abdominal appendages other than genitalia and cerci.

Subclass- Pterygota

Division: Exopterygota	Division: Endopterygota
Wings develop externally as bud.	Wings first develop as internal buds and then, they are projected out from wall of thorax.
Metamorphosis is incomplete.	Metamorphosis is complete.
Order: 1. Hemiptera (bugs) 2. Orthoptera (cockroach) 3. Phthyraptera (lice)	**Order:** 1. Diptera (flies) 2. Coleptera (beetles) 3. Hymenoptera (ants) 4. Siphonaptera (fleas)

Order: Diptera

Characters

1) They are called **true flies**.
2) It is one of the largest orders in the class Insecta, having more than 1, 20, 000 described species.
3) On thorax, there is only one pair of wing (**Di = two; ptera = wings**) i.e. Mesothoracic wing. Metathoracic pair of wings are modified into structures called "**Halters or balancers.**"

   Halter is a rod like structure having knob at distal end. During flight, this halter goes on vibrating @ 300 vibrations/sec. Its main function is to keep fly balanced during flying/flight.

4) One pair of compound eyes is present which is **dichoptic in female and holoptic in male.**

5) Larvae are **apodous** which is called **maggots.**

6) The order Diptera is divided into suborders, **Orthorrhapha** and **Cyclorrhapha**. These sub orders are distinguished morphologically by wing venation and structure of antennae.

Sub-Order

Orthorrhapha	**Cyclorrhapha**
1. Pupa of orthorrhaphan flies is of obtectate type. 2. Imago scoops out from pupa by muscling T- shaped. 3. Arista is absent. 4. Mandibles and 1st maxillae are present. 5. Ptilinium/ ptilinial suture is absent. 6. Abdominal segments are seven.	1. Pupa is coaractate type (puparium). 2. Imago makes circular opening on wall of puparium. 3. Arista is present. 4. Mandibles and 1st maxillae are absent. 5. Ptilinium is present which is **"Horse-shoe like"**. 6. Abdominal segments are less than seven, usually four.

Sub-Order: - Orthorrhapha

Series

Nematocera	**Brachycera**
Antennal segments are more than six in number.	Antennal segments are less than six.
Mandibles bite horizontally.	Mandibles bite vertically.
Famliy: a. Ceratopogonidae- Genus- *Culicoides* b. Simuliidae – Genus- *Simulium* c. Psychodidae– Genus–*Phlebotomus* d. Culicidae – Genus – i) *Culex* ii) *Anopheles* iii) *Aedes*	**Family:** **Tabanidae – Genus** a. *Tabanus* b. *Haematopota* c. *Chrysops* d. *Pangonia*

Suborder- Cyclorrhapha

Series

Aschiza	**Schizophora**		**Pupipara**
	Section: Calypterae	**Section: Acalypterae**	
Not of veterinary importance. It includes drone flies.	1. Ptilinium is distinct. 2. Squamma is large enough to cover halter. **Family:** 1. Muscidae 2. Glossinidae 3. Calliphoridae 4. Oestridae	1. Ptilinium is indistinct. 2. Squamma is small. It does not cover halter. **Family:** Gasterophilidae **Genus:** *Gasterophilus*	These are pupiparous insects. **Family:** Hippoboscidae **Genera:** **a.** *Hippobosca* **b.** *Pseudolynchia* **c.** *Mallophaga*

4

Order Diptera

Order: Diptera

Sub Order: Orthorrhapha

Series: Nematocera

Family: Ceratopogonidae

Genus: *Culicoides*

Species: *Culicoides oxystoma, C. imicola*

Common name: Biting midges or Biting gnats or punkies or No see-ums.

Hosts: Animals and man

Distribution: Worldwide

Morphology of fly

1. Size is 1-3 mm in length. They are the **smallest blood sucking flies. They can easily pass through mosquito nets.**
2. Head is spherical and has **piercing and sucking type of mouth parts.**
3. Antennae are 14/15 segmented. **It is plumose in male and pilose in female.**

   Note: Pilose means less hairy and hair are small in size. Plumose means long hair and large in numbers.
4. Thorax is slightly humped over the head.
5. **Wings are spotted (black spots are present)**, hairy and folded flat over abdomen during rest.

Anterior veins are stout and enclose two radial cells. Medial veins form two median forks.

Note: Space enclosed in wing veins are called cell.

Life cycle: Only females are blood suckers and host blood is essential for maturation of ovaries i.e. after blood meal, ovaries become matured and functional and thereafter, female start laying eggs. They lay 50-100 eggs in batches likewise; one female lays several hundred eggs during her life span. They lay eggs in stagnant water containing high organic matter i.e. **stagnant water containing high organic matter is the breeding place for *Culicoides* flies**. Flies deposit eggs on small object which are floating on water. Breeding places e.g. manure pits, blocked gutters, tree rice field. The eggs are banana shaped. The eggs hatch in about 3-4 days after deposition and larvae come out which is apodous and aquatic.

Larval body is made up of a head, three thoracic segment and nine abdominal segments (segments cannot be differentiated as thoracic and abdominal). Entire body is covered with thin spines and minute tubercles. On last abdominal segments, locomotory spines are present. Similarly, three gills are present. These larval stages fed upon small protozoa and protophyta (unicellular plants) present in breeding place. Larval stage lasts for 21 days (3 weeks). At the end, larvae migrate at the margin or periphery of breeding places where they moult to pupa. Pupal stage has head, thorax and abdominal segments. On thorax, two long respiratory trumpets are present. Entire body of pupa is again covered with spines and minute tubercles. On last abdominal segment of pupa, there are elongated spine with the help of which pupa holds itself and maintain erect position. Pupal stage is non- feeding resting stage. It lasts for five to seven days. Then it moults to adults and imago is emerged.

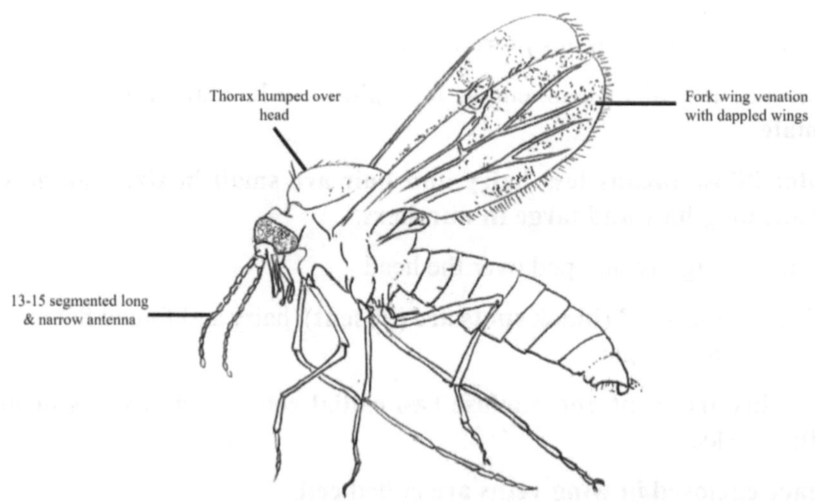

Figure 4.1. *Culicoides*

Habits of *Culicoides*

1. **Only females are blood suckers** and males feed on flower juices.
2. **They are active during twilight time**.ie. early in the morning and late in evening.
3. They usually do not enter into animal and human houses.
4. They attack different type of domesticated animal and human begins.
5. **They are very strong fliers. They can fly several kilometres at a stretch and can chase their prey also.**

Harmful Effcts

1. **Annoyance:** These flies are a serious source of irritation and annoyance to livestock. The head and neck are the main affected area by these flies. Bites are very painful and annoying i.e. animal goes on scratching and rubbing the affected parts and local inflammatory lesion are produced. These lesions may be invaded by secondary invasion and small micro abscesses may be produced.
2. **Allergic dermatitis:** Species which occur in Australia, cause allergic dermatitis in horses. This condition is known as **"Summer dermatitis, Queens land itch, Sweat itch or Sweet itch."** During this condition, when horses are first time exposed to bites, then there is no reaction. The first bite works as a sensitize dose. During the subsequent bites, severe allergic reactions take place in form of papules.
3. **Vector of pathogens:** *Culicoides* act as vectors of more than 50 arboviruses in various species of hosts. The fly transmits viral agents causing **blue tongue**, Eastern equine encephalitis, African horse sickness, Bovine ephemeral fever. It also acts as intermediate host for filarial worms belonging to genus *Onchocerca* (***Onchocerca cervicalis*** and ***Onchocerca gibsoni***) and genus *Dipetalonema* spp.

Control

a. **Elimination of breeding places:** It is an important step which if an undertaken carefully, then ninety percent prevention is possible. It can be done by providing proper drainage or irrigation to low lying areas.

b. **Spray of insecticides:** Insecticides (malathion, chlordane, chlorpyrophos etc.) should be applied which are having larvicidal effect. It should be sprayed on breeding ground and in and around animal houses.

Insecticides diluted in oil should be applied on breeding ground. For adult, insecticides should be sprayed particularly during day time on shrubs or dark places where adult hide during day time.

c. **Personal Protection:** By applying repellants on body of host.eg. Dimethyl phthalate, it is not economical since duration of action is only 5-6 hours. People in villages burn cow dung cake and resultant smoke has got repellent action on flies mainly in Assam and West Bengal (Kuki Areas).

Family: Psychodidae

Genus: *Phlebotomus*

Common name: Sand flies/ Owl midges/moth flies

Species: *Phlebotomus argentipes, P. sergenti, P. papatasi*

Host: Animals, man

Distribution: Warm and humid tropical region. In India, present in Rajasthan, eastern Uttar Pradesh, Bihar, Bengal, Orissa.

Morphological characters

1. Moth like flies.
2. Size near 5 mm in length.
3. **Piercing and sucking type of mouth parts present**.
4. Antenna does not show sexual dimorphism. Antennae are 12-16 segmented.
5. **Very long legs** are present.
6. **Wings are lanceolate in shape and held roof-like** over abdomen during rest.

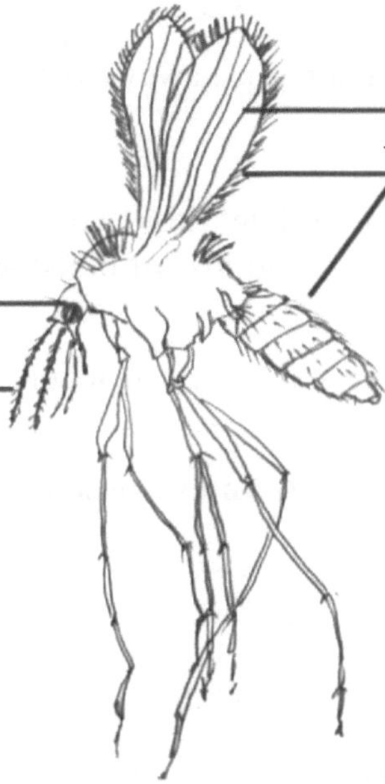
Lanceolate shaped wings
with parallel wing venation
Very smal and
hairy fly
Pominent eyes
16 segmented
long antenna

Figure 4.2. *Phlebotomus*

Life cycle

The female flies after its 1st blood meal lay about 40-50 eggs at a time in dark and moist places in cracks and crevices, below loose soil or under fallen leaves. Ovipositior of female is inserted into cracks and eggs are laid. These eggs have outer sticky layer with the help of which eggs are attached to walls of cracks and crevices. After 4-10 days, larvae hatch out from the eggs. Larva is apodous and larval body is divided into small head, three thoracic and nine abdominal segments. **They are caterpillar like with characteristic pinnate hair on body segments and pseudopods on ventral aspect of abdominal segments**. Entire larval body is covered with minute spines. On last abdominal segment, two pair of long, stiff bristles are present. These larval stages feed upon faeces of bird and lizzard and other organic matter and this stage lasts for 3-8 weeks, after which it moults to pupa. Pupal stage lasts for 5-6 days after which they moult to adult stages. Adult stage has short life span as they last for only 14 days.

Habits of *Phlebotomus*

1. **Only female are blood suckers.**
2. These flies are active during night time. i.e. **nocturnal in activity.**

3. These adult flies live for hardly 1-2 weeks.
4. They are weak flies; they cannot move away from breeding places.

Harmful Effects

1. These flies produce a painful bite (less painful in comparison to *Culicoides*) that cause irritation and loss of blood and a reduce weight gain.
2. Repeated bite causes hypersensitivity reaction and microabscess formation.
3. The fly act as **vector of cutaneous and visceral leishmaniosis.**

Family: Simuliidae

Genus: *Simulium*

Species: *Simulium indicum*

Common name: **Black flies /buffalo gnats**. In Himachal Pradesh, it is locally called **potu fly**.

Distribution: In Indian in sub-Himalayan region.

Morphological characters

1. They are black in colour. Body is covered with short golden or silvery hair.
2. Size is upto 5 mm.
3. **Thorax is humped over the head.**
4. **Short piercing and sucking type of proboscis.**
5. Antennae have 11 segments.
6. Wings are broad and have bristles on thick anterior veins.

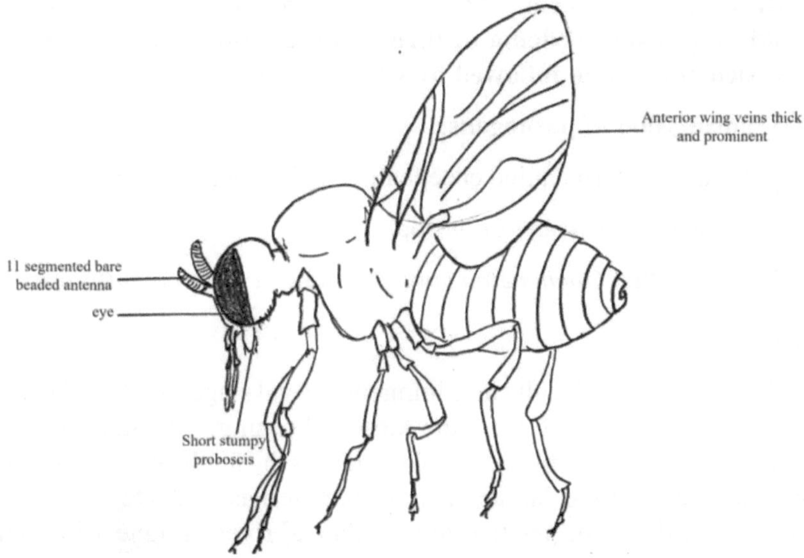

Figure 4.3. *Simulium* sp.

Life Cycle

Female inserts her ovipositor into the water and lay eggs. Eggs are deposited on stones or vegetation below the surface of running stream. Eggs hatch to release larvae which is cylindrical in shape and has posterior suckers armed with hooks for attachment to the objects. Near anterior extremity, on ventral surface there is an organ called **prolegs** which is arm like appendage with circlet of hooks. With the help of prolegs, larvae move. Larvae are carnivorous, moult six times and then **spin triangular cocoon** in which pupa develops. Pupa has one dorsal and one ventral respiratory tube which floats out of cocoon. Pupal stage lasts for 3-6 days then finally adult fly emerges.

Habits of black flies

1. Flies are active in the morning and evening and rest under the leaves during the day.
2. **Only females are blood sucker**

Harmful effects

1. **Annoyance and irritation**: Hovering and biting induce entomophobia in animals. Animals become restless, feeding is disturbed which ultimately results in production drop.

2. **Biting cause petechial haemorrhages particularly in areas of fine skin and cause oedema of throat and abdomen. Biting also causes vesicle formation followed by wart like papules on teat of cow.**
3. **Transmission of pathogens:**
    1. **Virus:** Eastern equine encephalitis and Vesicular stomatitis.
    2. **Protozoa:** *Leucocytozoon* spp.
    3. **Helminths**: *Onchocerca volvulus* and *Onchocerca gutturosa*

Control

Control is extremely difficult since immature larval stages are found in running water, often some distance from the farm or housing. The adult flies can fly over 5 km. The most common control method is the application of insecticides on breeding sites to kill larvae. This technique has been developed for the control of *Simulium* species that are vectors of river blindness in human in Africa, and entails the repeated application of insecticides to selected water sources at intervals throughout the year. Bush clearing is helpful to remove adult resting sites of flies.

Family: Culicidae

Mosquitoes comes under this family with more than 3000 described species. The family Culicidae is divided into two important sub families-

a. **Culicinae** includes *Culex* and *Aedes*

b. **Anophelinae** includes *Anopheles*

Hosts: Mammals, Birds and Reptiles

Morphological characters

1. They are small slender flies with long legs and size upto 5 mm in length.
2. **Antennae** are long, filamentous, segmented and **show sexual dimorphism i.e. plumose in male and pilose in female.**
3. Thorax is characteristically **wedge shaped**.
4. Wings are long, narrow and folded flat over abdomen when at rest. On wings 2nd and 4th wing veins are branched at tips. **Leaf like scales is present along the margin and on the veins.**

5. The mouthparts are conspicuous, forward-projecting, elongated proboscis adapted for piercing and sucking. Mouth parts comprise a long U-shaped fleshy labium containing paired maxillae, mandibles and a hypopharynx (carries a salivary duct). The labrum forms the roof of the proboscis. All the structures, except labium, enter the skin during feeding by the females, forming a tube through which blood is sucked. Males are non-parasitic and the maxillae and mandibles are reduced or absent. The maxillary palps of different species are variable in length and morphology.

Characters of different stage of genera *Anopheles*, *Culex* and *Aedes*

Stages	*Anopheles*	*Culex*	*Aedes*
Eggs	They lay eggs singly. Eggs are boat shaped with **lateral floats** on either side which helps to float on water.	Eggs are boat shaped and laid in **egg raft**. One raft contains around 300 eggs. Lateral float is absent.	Eggs are boat shaped, laid singly but without lateral float.
Larvae	1. Larva lies parallel to water surface. Palmate hair is present with the help of which it clings on to the surface of water. 2. **They are surface feeder** 3. **Siphon tube is absent.** 4. On 10th segment, tracheal gills are present.	1. Larva makes angle with surface water with **head hung down.** No palmate hair. 2. This is water feeder. 3. **Siphon tube is present on the fused 8th and 9th segments.** 4. On 10th segment, tracheal gills are present.	1. Similar to *Culex*. 2. **Tracheal gills** are well developed in so, it feeds on bottom of water.
Pupa	1. Comma shaped 2. Respiratory trumpets in pupal stages are short and board (funnel shaped).	1. Comma shaped 2. Respiratory trumpets are long and narrow.	Similar to *Culex*
Adult	1. **Female:** Maxillary Palps as long as proboscis and simple, not clubbed. **Male:** Palps as long as proboscis but clubbed. 2. During rest, abdomen directed away from resting surface i.e. **proboscis and abdomen are in straight line.** 3. Scutellum evenly curved. 4. No white marking.	1. **Female:** Maxillary palps are shorter than proboscis. **Male:** Maxillary palps as long as proboscis without swollen tip or not clubbed. 2. During rest, abdomen is directed towards the resting surface i.e. **proboscis and abdomen are at an angle giving humped back appearance.** 3. Scutellum is trilobed. 4. No white marking.	1. Similar to *Culex*. **2. White markings on joints of the legs**. Because of white strips they are commonly called **"tiger mosquitoes"**.

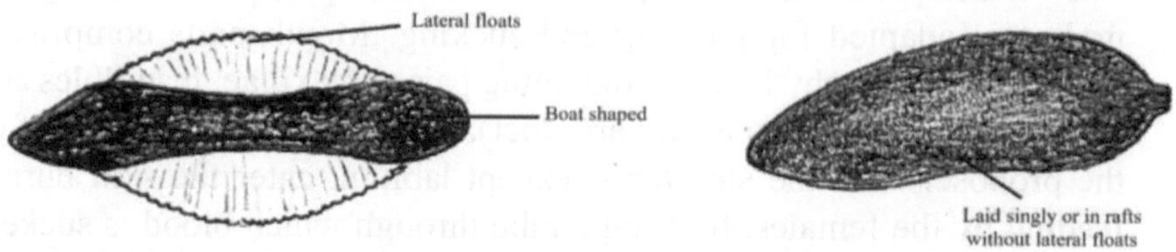

Figure 4.4. Egg of mosquito (a) *Anopheles* (b) *Culex*

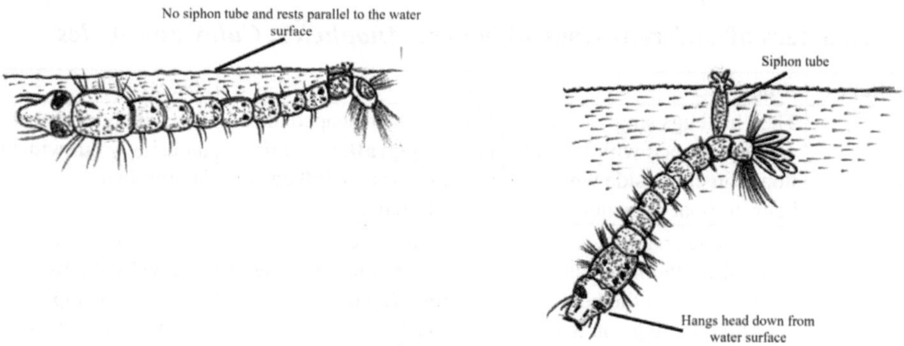

Figure 4.5. Larva of mosquito (a) *Anopheles* (b) *Culex*

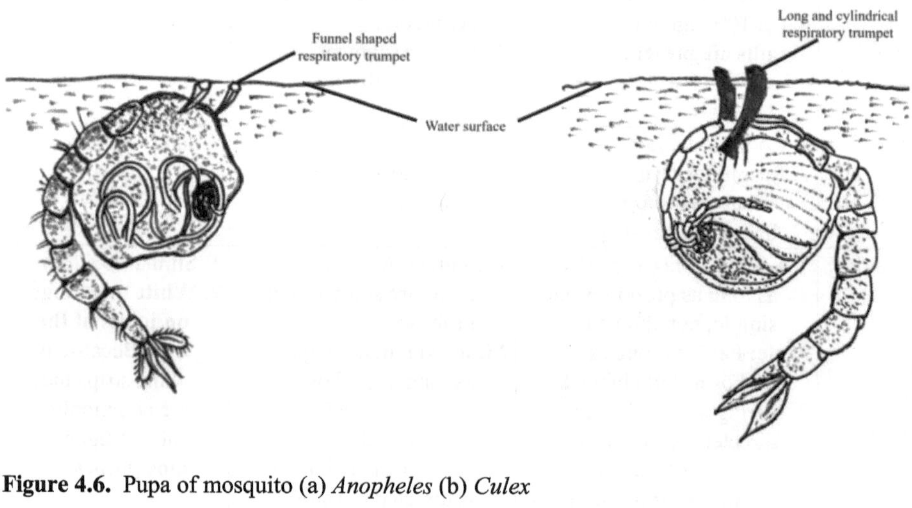

Figure 4.6. Pupa of mosquito (a) *Anopheles* (b) *Culex*

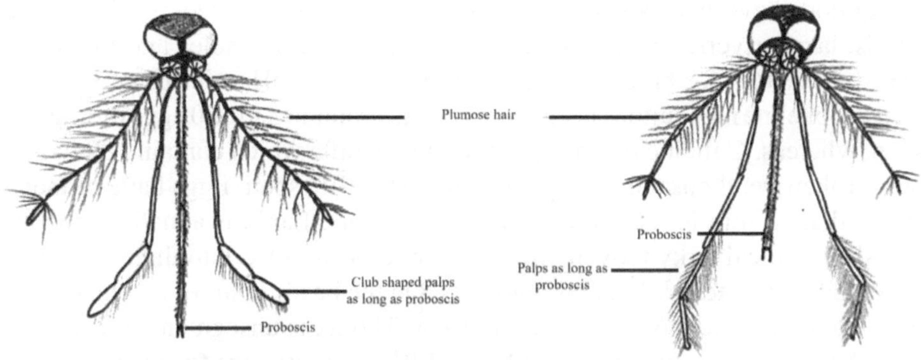

Figure 4.7. Mouth parts of *Anopheles* (a) Male (b) Female

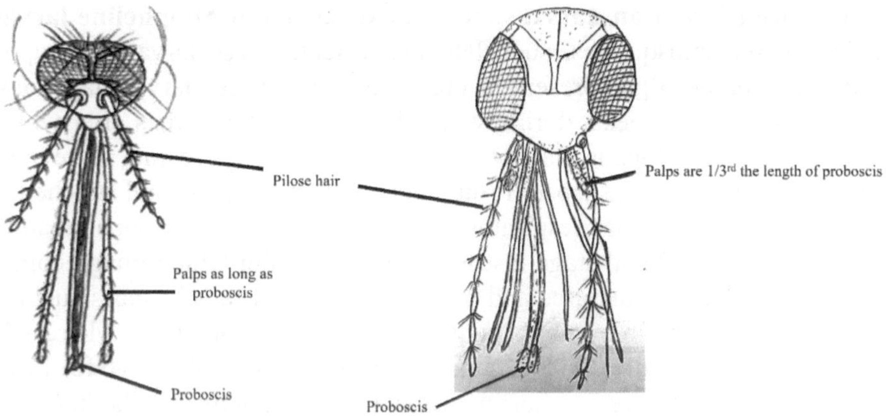

Figure 4.8. Mouth parts of *Culex* (a) Male (b) Female

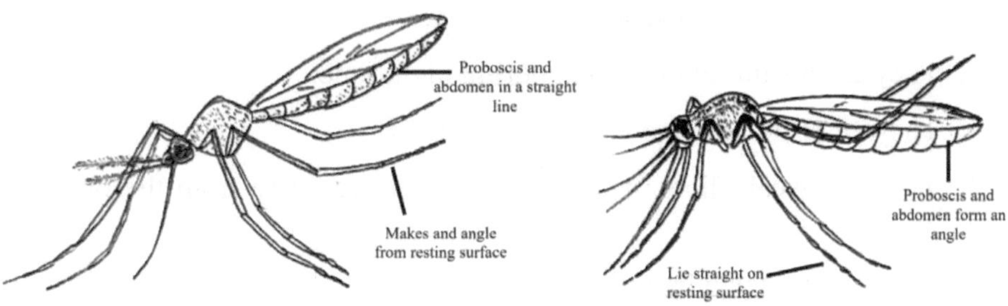

Figure 4.9 Adult mosquito (a) *Anopheles* (b) *Culex*

Life cycle

All species of mosquitoes have similar type of life cycle. Female after blood meal lay eggs in the water or on objects floating in water. Each species of mosquitoes have got its own requirement regarding its breeding places like ponds, lakes, rivers, streams, gutters, low line areas, bee holes and rice field. Deciding factors for breeding place are temperature, pH, microflora in water etc. Anopheline mosquitoes lay egg singly and around 75 to 150 eggs during life span, whereas, Culicine mosquitoes lay eggs in rafts which contain 100 to 300 eggs. Likewise, thousand of eggs are laid during life span. Eggs have rounded end and are 2 mm in length. Eggs hatch in 24 hrs. Larva is aquatic, apodous and show typical jerky movement. Larval body is divided into three parts i.e., head, thorax and ten abdominal segments. On the head, a pair of antennae, two eyes and brush like mouth parts are present. Thorax is unsegmented and bears hair. **Abdomen is segmented but 8th and 9th segments are fused. In case of Culicine larva on fused abdominal segments,** the siphon tube or respiratory trumpets are present. On last abdominal segments, gills are present. Plamate type hair **are present on dorsal surface of segments in Anopheline larvae** and in Culicine mosquitoes, such hair are absent. These larva feeds upon flagellates, ciliates, algae present at breeding place. These larval stages last for five days to two weeks, during which larva moult four times after which they moult to pupa which is non obtectate. It is non feeding, resting stage pupa which is aquatic, comma shaped. From dorsal aspect of thorax and attached to lateral stigmata, there arise respiratory trumpets through which pupa breathes at surface of water. Pupal stage last for 5 to 6 days after which imago comes out which in 24 hours matures and becomes adult and female starts sucking blood. In tropical or sub tropical country, there are 20 generations whereas in temperate regions, hardly 2 to 5 generation take place. Male flies live for 1 to 3 week and female also live for short time and die immediately after laying eggs.

Habits

1. Only female are blood suckers.
2. They are nocturnal i.e. attack during night time.
3. They enter into human and animal houses.
4. They are weak fliers, generally do not move away from the breeding places.
5. They are attracted by mild lights.

Harmful Effect

1. Allergic reaction takes place by the bite of mosquitoes.
2. Disease transmission:

a. **Human being:** Malaria caused by two species of *Plasmodium*, i.e. *Plasmodium vivax* and *Plasmodium falciparum*, Japanese encephalitis, dengue fever, yellow fever etc. Mosquitoes also acts as intermediate host for filarial worms called as "*Wuchereria bancroftii*" causing "Elephantiasis" in human beings.

b. **Animals:** Eastern equine encephalitis, *Plasmodium*, heart worm, *Setaria* etc.

Control

1. **Spray of insecticides:** Organophosphorous compound can be used like malathion @ 200g/ 100 sq.ft. Residual effect of 2-3 months.
2. **Mosquito repellants:** Mosquito coils are nothing but resin tapes which burn very slowly and, in these tapes, insecticides are incorporated.
3. **Light traps:** Mosquitoes are attracted towards light and in front of light electrical strings are placed so that gets trapped and electrocuted.
4. **Destruction of breeding ground:** Prevent accumulation of water. There should be proper drainage of water.
5. **Biological control of larval stages:** It is the control of harmful pest by using their natural enemies.

   a. **Fish rearing**: *Gambusia* fish which is larvivorous that eats larvae of mosquitoes.

   b. **Plants**

   i. **Chara:** It produces more oxygen which is detrimental to larval stage.

   ii. ***Urticularia*:** The networks of branches of *Urticularia* trap larval and pupal stage of mosquitoes.

   iii. ***Lymna*:** The very broad leaves of this plant cover the surface of water so adult cannot emerge out and die due to asphyxia.

6. **Genetic control of mosquito**

Sterile male technique: Males are made sterile by using chemical or irradiation. These males are let loose in environment. These sterile males outcompete fertile males for fertilizing females, hence mosquito population is reduced.

Incompatible interbreeding: Breeding between two species of mosquitoes i.e. *Anopheles* and *Culex* and *Anopheles* and *Aedes* results in sterile progeny.

Transgenic mosquitoes: Mosquitoes are being genetically modified in the lab either to suppress mosquito population or to stop the development of parasites in them. Some mosquitoes have been incorporated with self limiting genes which when passed to mosquitoes offsprings affects their normal process. These affected offsprings do not survive to adulthood. Also, genetic modification is being done in mosquitoes which cause release of compounds in their gut that stunt the growth and development of parasites like *Plasmodium*.

Order: Diptera

Sub- Order: Orthoprhapha

Series: Brachycera

Brachycera are a major series of the order Diptera with around 120 families. The most discriminate characteristic of Brachycera is reduced antenna segmentation.

Family: Tabanidae

Tabanidae is one of the largest families of order Diptera, including approximately 8000 species divided into 30 genera (horse flies), *Haematopota* (clegs), *Chrysops* (deer flies) and *Pangonia* are the genera of major veterinary importance.

Morphological characters

1. They are large, robust flies with strong wings.
2. Eyes are large, dichoptic in female and holoptic in male.
3. **Antennae are three segmented, terminal segment is largest and has annulations.**
4. Fourth longitudinal wing vein branches to enclose space called **discal or hexagonal cell.**
5. Mandibles are strong and bite horizontally. **It cut skin like scissors and blood oozes out.** Mouth part is cutting and sponging type as **labella has pseudotracheal membrane** with the help of which it sponges the oozed-out blood.

Genera

***Tabanus*- Horse fly or breeze fly**

***Haemotopota* – clegs**

***Chrysops* - deer fly**

Pangonia

Difference between genera *Tabanus* (horse flies), *Haematopota* (clegs), *Chrysops* (deer flies) and *Pangonia*

Character	*Tabanus*	*Haematopota*	*Chrysops*	*Pangonia*
Mouth	Short, proboscis hang downwards.	Short, proboscis hang downwards.	Long, proboscis hang downwards.	Very long, proboscis is projected in forward direction.
Antennae	1st and 2nd segments are small and 3rd big. Third segment has **tooth like projection at its basal part** and has **four annulations.**	1st and 3rd are big and 2nd is small. 3rd segment bears **three annulations.**	All the segments are equally big. 3rd segment bears **four annulations.**	All segments are big. 3rd segment bears **6-7 annulations.**
Eyes	Non metallic colour.	Non metallic colour.	Metallic colour	Non metallic colour.
Wings	**Clear**	Wings has **scroll like mottling.**	**Dark band extending from anterior margin to posterior margin** of wings in the middle.	Brownish band or spots.

Life cycle

Female, after first blood meal lay around 500-600 eggs on the leaves or objects which are overhanging on the water surface particularly branches of tree. Eggs are 2 mm long, spindle shaped; creamish white when freshly laid, later becomes dark brown at time of hatching. These larvae immediately drop down in water as these larvae are aquatic. Larva can also survive at muddy place.

Larvae are 1-6 cm in length. It has cephalic region followed by 11 segments. On cephalic region, antennae are present. On each segment, 8 fleshy tubercles are present. On the second last segment, there is siphon tube. These larvae are carnivorous in nature. They feed upon young crustacean. Laval stage last for 2-3 months at the end of which larvae migrate to margin of ponds towards drier part and moult to pupa. Pupa is segmented and is obtectate type. Entire pupal body is covered with long hair. Pupal stage lasts for 10-19 days and then an imago comes out. Under favourable conditions, whole life cycle takes 4-5 months to complete. There are 2 -3 generations of *Tabanus* per year particularly in tropical country.

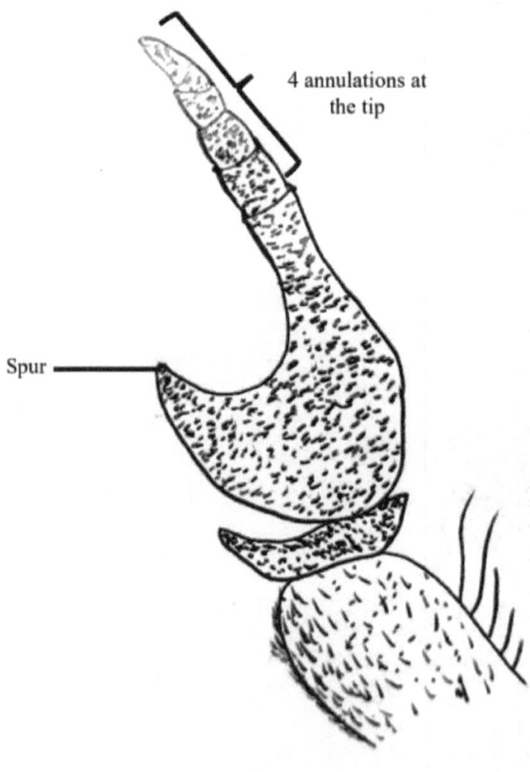

Figure 4.10. Antennae of *Tabanus*

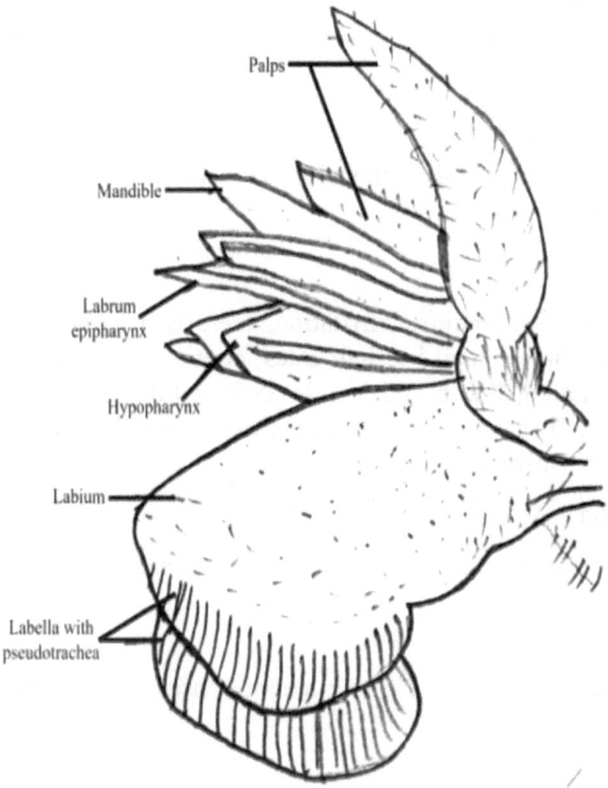

Figure 4.11. Mouth Parts of *Tabanus*

Habit of *Tabanus*

1. **Only females are blood sucker** and males thrive on vegetable matter, fruit etc.

2. ***Tabanus* are active during day time, particularly when there is bright sunshine.**

3. They do not enter into animal houses, but attack the animal standing in open, they particularly attack large animals and they bite on neck region, lower side of abdomen and legs.

4. They **feed intermittently** as their feeding is disturbed due to sudden movement of animal which is caused by painful bite of *Tabanus*. They suck around 0.5 ml of blood. But during these, they make several cut injuries on skin. **Intermittent feeding is important in disease transmission,** since when feeding gets disturbed by animal movement,

then fly sits on adjacent animals which is idle. Like wise it bites many animals in the vicinity. So, if the fly is infected, it transmits infection particularly of surra to several animals.

5. **They feed once in 2-3 days.**
6. They are very strong flyers and **fly generally very close to surface of water taking occasional dips.**

Harmful Effect

- **Painful bite:** Bites are very painful, irritation, there is a great blood loss because wounds that created by their bites, continue to bleed for some time. It is estimated that, blood loss is 25-75 ml/day in heavily infected area and animal suffer from anaemia. Wounds may be infected with bacteria or screw worm myiasis.
- **Disease transmission**

i. **Protozoan diseases:** *Tabanus* transmit very important haemoprotozoan disease "Surra" caused by *Trypanosoma evansi*. Tabanus also transmit *Trypanosoma equinum*, *Trypanosoma theileri,*

ii. **Virus:** Equine infectious anaemia, Bovine leucosis virus, Hog cholera virus.

iii. **Bacteria:** *Bacillus anthracis*

iv. **Rickettsials:** *Anaplasma*

v. **Nematodes**: Loa loa, *Elaephora schneideri*

Control

- **Destruction of breeding place:** Branches of trees hanging on water should be eliminated.
- Providing drainage to low lying area where water is not used by humans.
- Since flies have habit of skimming over water and take occasional dips, pouring of kerosene oil onto water kills the adult fly when they take dips.
- Personal protection by using repellents, fly proof net etc.
- Use of carbon dioxide baited traps or light traps.

Order: Diptera

Sub Order: Cyclorrhapha

Character

1. Pupa is coarctate type.
2. Ptilinium is present, they make circular slit on wall of puparium when imago comes out.
3. Arista is present.
4. Mandible and maxillae are absent.
5. Abdominal segment are less than seven usually four.

Series: Schizophora

Section: Calypterae and Acalypterae

Calypterae	Acalypterae
Squamae are well developed and halters are concealed.	Squamae small but halters are not concealed.
Thorax has distinct transverse sutures.	Thorax without distinct transverse sutures.

Section: Calypterae

Family: Muscidae

Character

This family comprises of many biting and non-biting genera. The non biting genera is referred as nuisance flies. These flies are responsible for 'fly-worry' in livestock. These flies act as vectors of various bacterial, helminth and protozoal organisms. The major genera of veterinary importance include *Musca* (house flies and related flies), *Stomoxys* (stable fly), *Haematobia* (horn flies, buffalo flies) and *Hydrotaea* (sweat and head flies). The Importnt characters is absence of hypopleural bristles.

Differential characters of *Musca* and *Stomoxys* spp.

Character	*Musca*	*Stomoxys*
Species	*Musca domestica* (house fly) *Musca autumnalis* (face fly)	*Stomoxys calcitrans* (Stable fly)
Proboscis	**Lapping and sponging type**. Proboscis is retractile and labella have pseuotrachea which is used to suck the fluid.	**Cutting and sucking type**. Proboscis is non retractile and it is **bayonet shaped.** Labella has teeth.

Character	*Musca*	*Stomoxys*
Arista	**Bilaterally plumosed**	**Unilaterally plumosed**. Hair is present on dorsal side only.
Thorax	Four dark longitudinal stripes are present on dorsal aspect of thorax which extends up to the posterior border of the scutum.	Four dark longitudinal stripes are present but lateral one does not reach upto the scutum.
Abdomen	Median dark longitudinal stripes are present which diffuse on the fourth segment.	Abdomen is shorter and broader than housefly. There are three dark spots on each of second and third segments.
Wings	**Fourth longitudinal wing vein (M_{1+2}) sharply turns upwards making apical cell (R5) narrow.**	**Fourth longitudinal wing vein (M_{1+2}) gently turns upwards making apical cell (R5) wide open**
Eggs	Lay around 100-150 eggs at a time upto total of 1000 eggs.	Lay around 25-50 eggs at a time upto total of 800 eggs.
Larvae	Stigmal plates are **'D'** shaped. In each stigma plates, **three 'M' shaped** slits are present. Distance between two stigmal plates are narrower.	Stigmal plates are triangular in shaped. In each stigma plates, **three 'S'** shaped slits are present. Distance between two stigmal plates are wider.

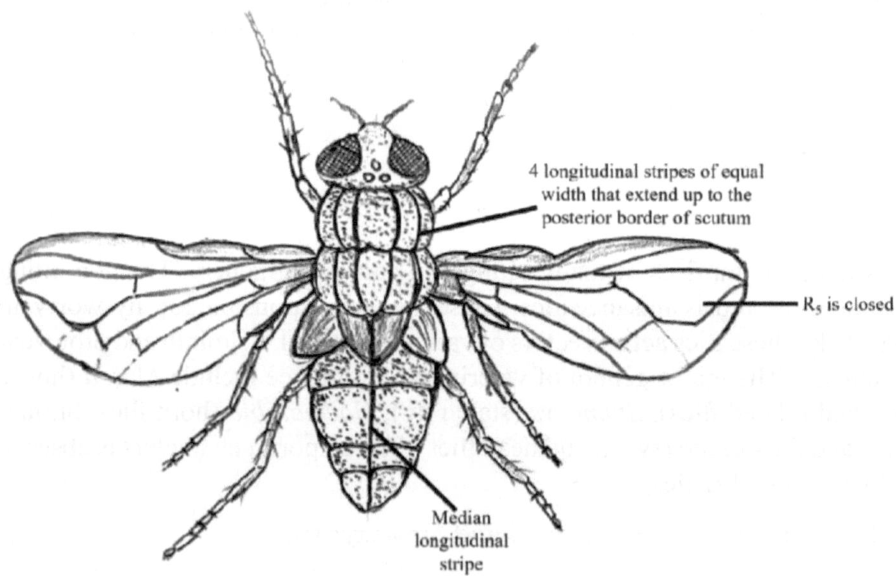

Figure 4.12. *Musca domestica* (Adult)

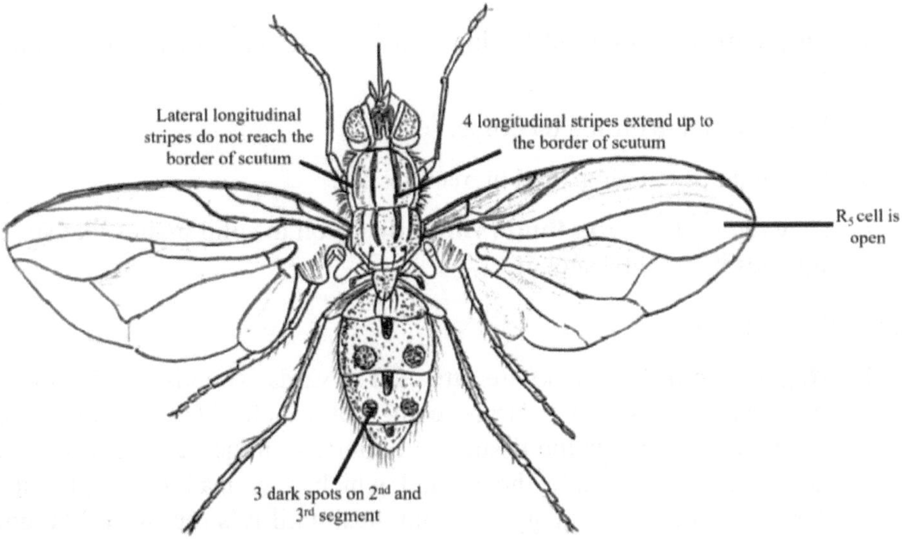

Figure 4.13. *Stomoxys* (Adult)

Musca spp.

Life cycle: Female flies live for 6-8 weeks and after proteinaceous meal, they start laying eggs. They are not blood suckers only they feed on blood. One female lay around 1000 eggs during her life span and at a time they deposit around 100-150 eggs on dung or manure. Similarly, they can also deposit egg on wound and other decomposing organic matter. Eggs are 1 mm creamy white in colour and **on dorsal side of eggs there are 2 longitudinal ribs like depression**. These eggs hatch during 12- 36 hours and larvae come out. Larva is apodous, 10- 12 mm in length. Anterior end is narrow and posterior end is comparatively broad on which stigmal plates are present. **At anterior end, a pair of oral hooks are present attached to internal cephalopharyngeal skeleton,** which are composed of darkly pigmented chitin. These larval stages last for 3-7 days after they migrate out of breeding places and penetrates into superficial layer of soil, where they moult to pupa. Pupa is coarctate type i.e., skin of last larva is retained on pupa in form of puparium. Pupa of *Musca* is barrel shaped, dark down in colour last for 14-28 days at the end of which imago comes out. The female flies become mature in 10-14 days and start laying eggs.

Habits of House fly

1. Only female takes food having proteins and sugar meal from animal matter.
2. They are active during day time.
3. They enter into animal and human houses.
4. They regurgitate **crop fluid (Vomit drop)** on to solid matter like sugar, liquefies it and then suck it.

Harmful Effects

1. **Maggot wound:** Female are attracted towards wounds and lays eggs there. Eggs hatches and larvae come out which aided by oral hooks penetrate deep inside the tissues and interfere in the healing of wound. Adult also contaminate the wound which may lead to suppuration. Wound infected with maggots do not heal until it is removed. Maggots are either removed manually using forceps or mixture of chloroform and terpentine oil (1: 1) is topically poured over the wound. After some time, remove the maggots.
2. **Disease transmission:** House fly has the habit of frequent regurgitation of crop fluid and defaecating at frequent interval which plays significant role in mechanical transmission of number of diseases.
   i. **Bacterial diseases:** Cholera *(Vibrio cholera),* Typhoid *(Salmonella typhimurium)*, Anthrax (*Bacillus anthracis*).
   ii. **Viral diseases:** Poliomyelitis.
   iii. **Protozoan diseases:** Amoebiasis, Giardiasis
   iv. **Helminths:** They act as intermediate host for *Habronema megastoma, Habronema muscae, Raillietina, Stephanofilaria, Parafilaria bovicola* and *Thelazia* species.

Control

Elimination of breeding place: Dung of different animal, decaying vegetable material, bedding material like hay which is soiled with urine. Hence these things may be disposed off hygienically. In addition to reduce the population of fly in that particular area, spraying of insecticide is useful.

Stomoxys calcitrans (stable fly)

Life cycle: Stable fly prefers to lay eggs on decaying matter like straw, hay, vegetables especially when contaminated with urine. A female lays 25-50 eggs at a time. Eggs 1 mm in length are dirty white to yellow and has longitudinal groove on one side. Eggs hatch in 1-4 days to give larvae which feed on vegetable matter. Larvae stage lasts for 14-24 days and pupa stage duration is 6-9 days. Life cycle completes in about one month.

Habits

1. **Both male and female are blood suckers.**
2. They prefer fairly strong light, not seen in dark stable or house.

Harmful Effects

1. Disease transmission

Protozoan: *Trypanososma*

Helminths: Intermediate host for *Habronema majus*

Other muscid flies

***a. Hydrotaea irritans* (head fly)**

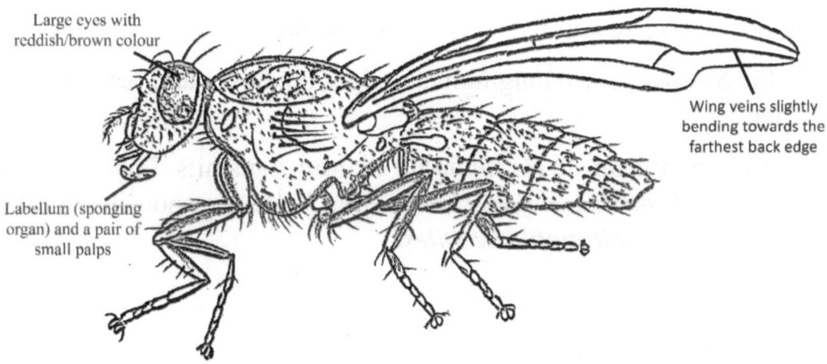

Figure 4.14. *Hydrotaea irritans*

Characters

1. **Non biting fly.**
2. 4-7 mm in length.
3. Thorax is black with grey patches and abdomen is olive green and wing base are orange yellow.

b. Haematobia

i. ***Haematobia exigua* (Buffalo fly)**
ii. ***Haematobia irritans* (Horn fly)**

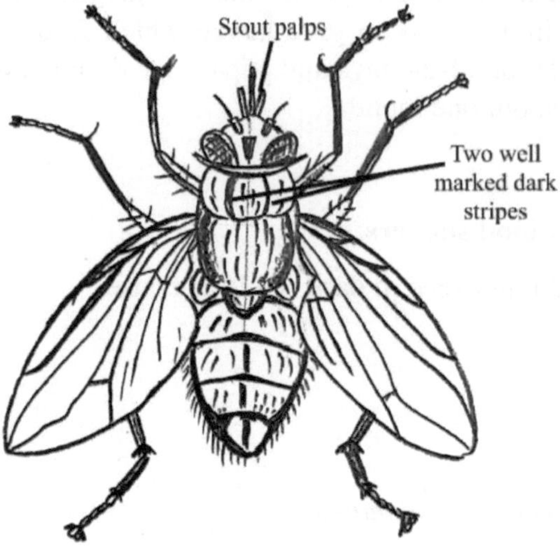

Figure 4.15. *Haematobia* spp.

Characters and significance

1. Biting fly, both male and female are blood suckers.
2. Resemble *Stomoxys*, two longitudinal stripes on thorax and few spots on abdomen.
3. Pathogenic significance: ***Haematobia exigua*** transmits ***Trypanosoma evansi*** and ***Habronema majus***. ***Haematobia irritans*** responsible for the transmission of ***Stephanofilaria stilesi.***

Family Glossinidae

Genus: *Glossina* (tse tse fly)

The species and eight subspecies of tsetse fly are demonstrated that can be divided into three groups on the basis of different habits and requirements. *Glossina palpalis* group are the riverine species that feed primarily on reptiles and ungulates blood. Flies of the group of *G. morsitans* are savannah and dry thorn-bush species and feed mainly on large animals. Members of the group *G. fusca* found in the rainforest, mainly dense shade and riverine thickets.

Distribution: Restricted to sub-Saharan Africa. Not found in India.

Characters

1. **Blood sucking flies** - both sexes feed exclusively on the blood of vertebrates.

2. **They are pupiparous flies.**
3. **Wings has hatchet or cleaver shaped** cells or axe shape like cell (M_2 cell).
4. **Transmits: *Trypanosoma* in man and animals.**

Breeding of *Glossina* generally reported throughout the year, with peak fly numbers found at the end of the rainy season. The longevity of adult flies in nature is variable, ranging from a few days to several months.

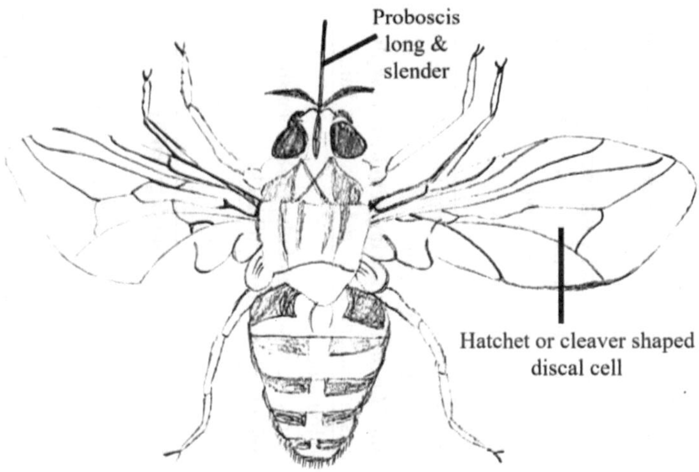

Figure 4.16. *Glossina* sp. (Adult)

Family: Calliphoridae

The flies under this family are, known as blowflies. It is a large family, having more than 1000 species divided into 150 genera. The various species of these flies are responsible for the infestation of the tissues of a living vertebrate host called traumatic myiasis.

Characters

1. They have well developed hypopleural bristles.
2. Mouth parts are adopted for lapping purpose.
3. The adult flies are non-parasitic while their larval stages living in tissues of different animals or human being are parasitic.
4. They are oviparous.

Two Subfamily

A. Calliphorinae

B. Sarcophaginae

A. Subfamily: Calliphorinae

Genus /Species	Common name	Characters	Nature of fly
Lucilia serricata and *L. cuprina*	Green bottle or copper bottle fly	1. 8-10 mm long. 2. **They are metallic green or bronze in colour**. 3. Eyes are brownish red. 4. Large bristles on thorax and abdomen. 5. **Like *Musca*, fourth wing vein bent sharply**. 6. *L. serricata* legs are black whereas in *L. cuprina*, femora of first pair of legs are bright green. 6. **Non blood suckers**.	Blow fly/facultative fly Blow fly/facultative fly
Calliphora	Blue bottle fly	1. Large stoutly built fly, 12mm long. 2. **Metallic blue** in colour. 3. **Like *Musca*, fourth wing vein bent sharply.** 4. Eyes are red and genae red with black hair.	
Phormia	Black blow fly	1. 6-11mm long. 2. Thorax black with **metallic blue green sheen.** 3. **Abdomen blue-green to black.**	
Chrysomyia albicepes, C. micropogon, C. ruffifacies	Sheep blow fly of Australia	-	
Chrysomyia bezziana	Old world screw worm fly	1. **Medium sized stout bluish green fly**. 2. Face is orange yellow. 3. Four black stripes on the prescutum are present.	Screw worm/ Obligatory fly
Cochliomyia (*Callitroga*) *hominivorax*			Screw worm/ Obligatory fly
Cordylobia anthropophaga	Tumbu fly or skin maggot fly	Not in India. Seen in Africa. Mostly affect man, dogs, monkey.	Facultative fly

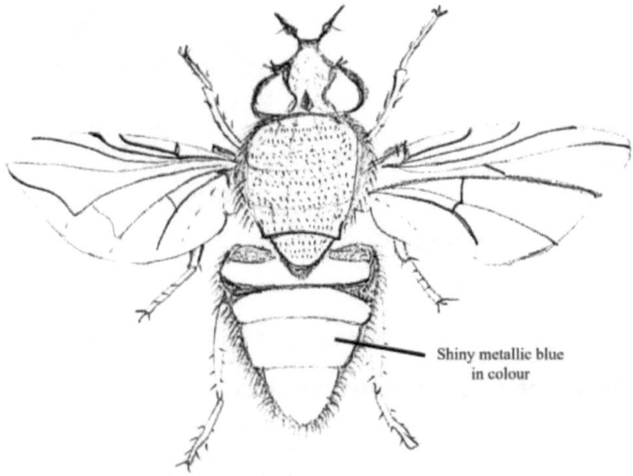

Figure 4.17. *Calliphora* fly (Adult)

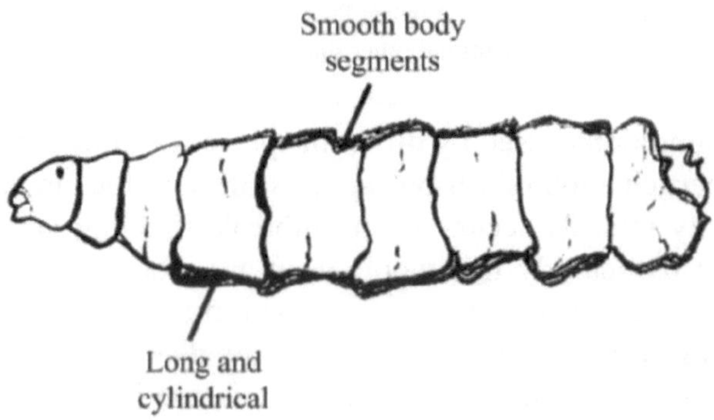

Figure 4.18. *Lucilia* larva

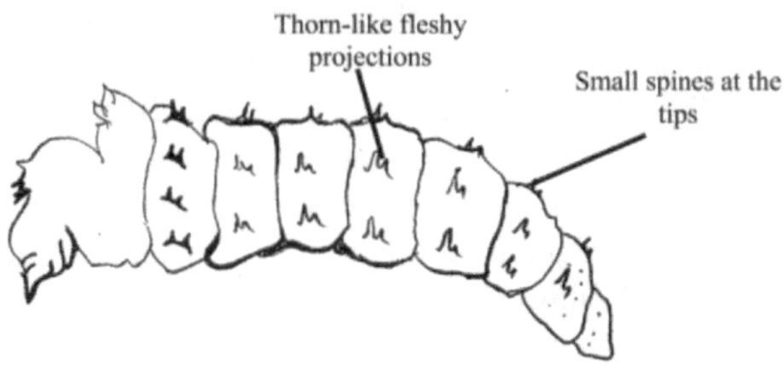

Figure 4.19. *Chrysomyia* larva

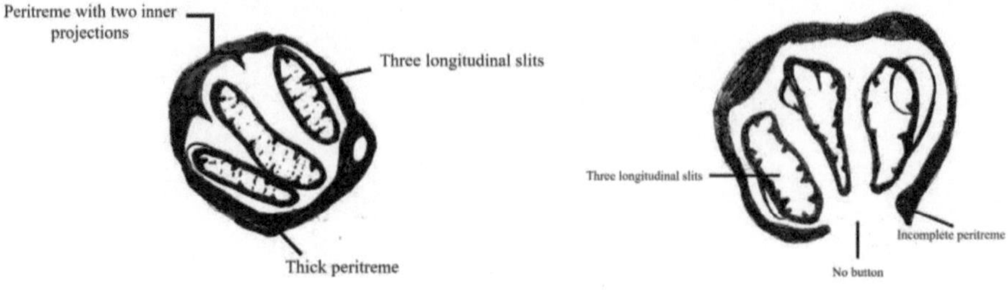

Figure 4.20. Spiracles of **(a)** *Calliphora* larva **(b)** *Chrysomyia* larva

Difference in larvae of blow flies and screw worm flies

Blow fly larave	Screw-worm fly larvae
Larvae are smooth without spines.	Larvae of screw-worm flies have bands of spines on each segment (encircling) giving typical appearance of cork-screw. Hence called screw-worm flies.
Larvae are responsible for causing cutaneous myiasis or Blow fly myiasis or Strike in sheep.	Larvae of screw worm flies cause screw worm myiasis in animal other than sheep.

Blow flies myiasis: It is a condition caused by different species of blow flies. This condition caused by participation of various species of blow flies in an organized way. This blow fly myiasis occurs as an outbreak affecting large number of sheep at a time; particularly fine wool sheep are more severely affected. Similarly in heavily infected cases, there may be mortality. **Disease condition in sheep which are infected with larvae of blow flies are called as ''Strike''** and affected animal is called **'struck'.** This disease is a severe problem in Australia, heavily affecting sheep productivity. However, few outbreaks have been recorded in North India.

Life cycle of blow flies: Adult flies live for very short period hardly for one month during which they take protein rich food. These proteinaceous foods are required for egg deposition. They lay 30-50 eggs at a time and about 2000-3000 eggs during her life span. These flies lay eggs on decomposing animal matter like carcass as well as on body of the host. These eggs hatch within 3-8 hours and larva undergoes two subsequent moults to form 3rd stage larvae. Third stage larvae are formed within 19 days depending on climatic condition. Subsequently third stage larvae drop down from animal body or carcass on the soil and then they penetrate in superficial layers of soil for pupation. Pupal stage lasts for 3-6 days and adult flies come out from pupa. When climatic conditions are suitable i.e., prolonged wet weather (temperature 27-33°C), life cycle can be completed within 7-8 days. Likewise, there may be even 7-8 generations of blow flies in a season. Apart from climatic conditions, availability of food and degree of decomposition of carcass or wound also influence the life cycle. Larvae of blow flies are smooth and resemble in morphology with larvae of *Musca* but they can be differentiated on basis of posterior spiracles. There are 2 types of larvae of blow flies: hairy larva and smooth larva. Hairy larva has stiff hair on body and in smooth larva hair is absent.

Epizootiology or Epidemiology of Blow Fly Myiasis

Factor influencing the occurrence of blow flies myiasis can be divided into two categories: 1. Factors determining the occurrence of flies:

a) **Season:** Different species of blow flies are adapted to different climatic condition so they occur in particular season and this season is called as "fly season." Humidity and temperature influence the occurrence of flies. Likewise in India, there are two fly seasons 1) February to March, 2) October to November. All the species of blow flies do not occur simultaneously neither in actual fly season nor throughout the season. But there are successive over lapping waves in the occurrences of blow flies.

b) **Availability of food for adults as well as for larval stages:** Different species of blow flies prefer carcass or wound at different stages of decomposition. Depending upon availability of food in a fly season, at a particular period only those species of blow flies will occur more in nature for which adequate suitable food is available. Depending on this utilization of feeding places, blow flies can be divided as:

   i) **Primary blow flies:** Prefer carcass wound at an early stage of decomposition. These primary flies initiate the myiasis. e.g. *Lucilia, Calliphora* and *Phormia.*

   ii) **Secondary blow flies:** Deposit eggs on carcass or wound at subsequent stages of decomposition or autolysis or even liquefaction. So, larvae of secondary flies extend the myiasis. In other words, these secondary flies breed on sheep which are already struck by primary flies. Thus, they extend myiasis. e.g. *Chrysomyia, Sarcophaga* and some species of *Calliphora.*

   iii) **Tertiary blow flies:** These flies arrive at last stage and further extend the damage. They are accidental in performance. e.g. *Musca.*

Out of these, primary flies are more important because they initiate myiasis by depositing eggs on body of sheep. When primary flies feed on fresh wounds, larvae of primary flies bring about certain changes in wound which attracted secondary flies. Primary flies make the wounds more suitable for secondary and tertiary flies. Larvae of secondary flies are very strong and they eat the larvae of primary flies. Similarly tertiary fly larvae remove larvae of secondary flies.

2. Factors determining the susceptibility of the host:

a) Inherent factors: Mainly due to "Faulty Body Confirmations"

Example:

(1) **Narrow breech:** Two tuber ischii bones when located very close to each other, then skin of this region is wrinkled and thrown in folds. In these folds, faeces and urine go on accumulating which results into continuous irritation and finally inflammation sets in. As a result, there is exudation and typical smell which attract the primary flies.

(2) **Narrow preputial sheath:** In certain breeds of sheep, preputial opening is very small as a result, urine goes on dripping from prepuce, so wool of adjacent area becomes wet and similar kinds of reaction takes place.

(3) **Narrow poll:** Horns are located very close to each other in certain breeds of sheep, so skin of forehead region is thrown into microfolds. In these folds, sweat goes on accumulating and inflammation sets in. This again attracts primary flies.

b. Temporary factors

i. **Open wounds on body of sheep:** presence of wounds on the body attract the flies.

ii. **Diarrhoea in animals:** Animals suffering from diarrhoea, soil the body parts which again creates medium for bacterial multiplication which subsequently results in inflammation and itching.

iii. **Prolonged wet weather:** Prolonged wet weather increase moisture on the body of animal which creates conducive environment for bacterial growth.

Pathogensis: Presence of wound or discharge from wounds attracts the flies. The flies deposit eggs in wounds and myiasis occurs. Wool absorbs moisture and presence of yolk material creates ideal medium for the growth of bacteria. As a result, inflammation occurs. Eggs hatch and larva comes out. These primary larvae feed upon the exudate and yolk material and also produced proteolytic enzymes. As a result, liquefaction of adjacent tissues takes place.

When there is suppuration, secondary flies come and breed and extend myiasis as larvae of secondary flies penetrate deep in wounds and large wounds are produced on body, such wounds do not heal because of migration of larval stages. Extensively infected sheep may die, so during severe outbreaks there is mortality. Sheeps are affected with blow fly larvae most frequently in the breech **(breech strike or crutch strike)** and around the tail **(tail strike).** In rams, preputial sheath with narrow openings is also affected **(pizzle strike).**

Symptoms

1. Infected sheep become dull and anorectic.
2. As a result of cutaneous myiasis, they try to rub affected part against hard objects and further injure its body.
3. Breakage and discolouration of wool with bad smell **(fleece rot).**
4. In case of septicaemia, increase of temperature and pulse rate.

Diagnosis

1. Presence of larvae in wounds. Larvae are deeply embedded in wounds in which only posterior ends are visible.

Treatment: Wool of affected part should be clipped off and exposed skin should be dressed with insecticide ointment. Similarly, larvae should be removed from wound. Deeply seated larvae can be removed by application of chloroform or Nilgiri oil. Larvae coming out can be removed.

Prevention

a. Proper dressing of wounds.
b. Crutching the wool from around the tail and in the breech. This promotes dryness in the region.
c. Surgical removal of breech folds.
d. Treat diarrhoea cases.
e. Postpone minor surgical operation during rainy season.
f. Application of insecticides during fly season on body of hosts and premises.
g. Use of light traps to control fly population.
h. Proper disposal of carcass.
i. Selective breeding in order to rectify faulty body conformations.

B. Subfamily: Sarcophaginae

Most species under this sub family are of no veterinary importance. They breed on carrion and other decomposing organic matter. *Wohlfahrtia* is the principal genus which act as important agents of myiasis in animals. Members of the genus *Sarcophaga* may occasionally infest on wounds. *Sarcophaga haemorrhoidalis* is the more widely distributed species.

Characters

1. They are called **'flesh flies'** also called **carrion flies**
2. Medium to large sized flies with light or dark grey in colour.
3. **Arista is plumose to about its middle but bare in the distal portion.**
4. Thorax has three longitudinal dark stripes whereas **abdomen is chequered dark and grey**.
5. **They are larviparous.**

Genus/Species

i. ***Sarcophaga dux:*** Common in India. Lay larvae in skin lesions of animals.

ii. ***Wohlfahrtia magnifica***: It is called **old world flesh fly.** Seen in West Asia.

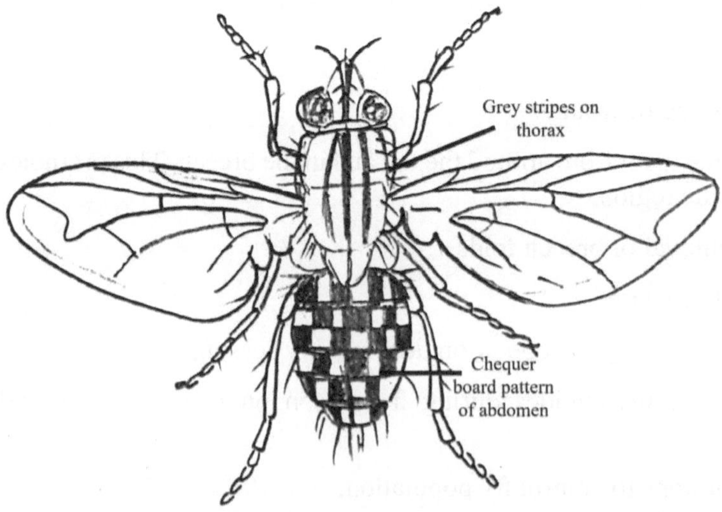

Figure 4.21. *Sarcophaga* (Adult)

Family: Oestridae (Bot fly)

The flies under this family are large and usually hairy. The larvae are obligatory parasites of animals. The adults have primitive non-functional mouthparts. However, the larvae spend their entire period of larval growth and development feeding within their vertebrate hosts, causing nasopharyngeal, digestive tract or dermal–furuncular myiasis. The larvae are characterised by posterior spiracular plates containing numerous small pores.

Characters

1. Members of this family are medium size with mouth part lapping type.
2. Due to rudimentary mouth part, adult do not feed at all.
3. Adult has short life span.
4. Hypopleural bristles are present.
5. **Larval stage is parasitic whereas adults are free living.**
6. They cause **obligatory myiasis**.
7. They are highly **host specific**.

Genera of importance are (a) *Oestrus* (b) *Hypoderma*

Genus: *Oestrus*

Species: *Oestrus ovis*

Host: Sheep and goat. Man gets accidentally affected.

Common name: Sheep nasal fly/sheep nasal bot fly

Morphological characters

1. Fly is medium size, 12-14mm in length.
2. They are greyish in colour and whole body is covered with brown coloured hair. Black spots are present on thorax and abdomen.
3. Antennae have bare arista.
4. **Fly is larviparous/viviparous.**

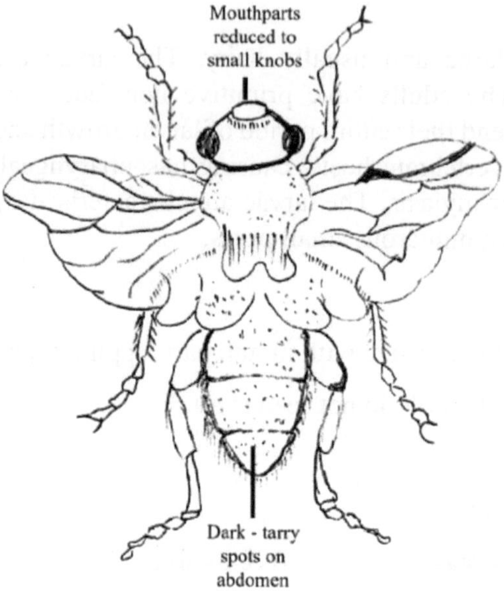

Figure 4.22. *Oestrus ovis* (Adult)

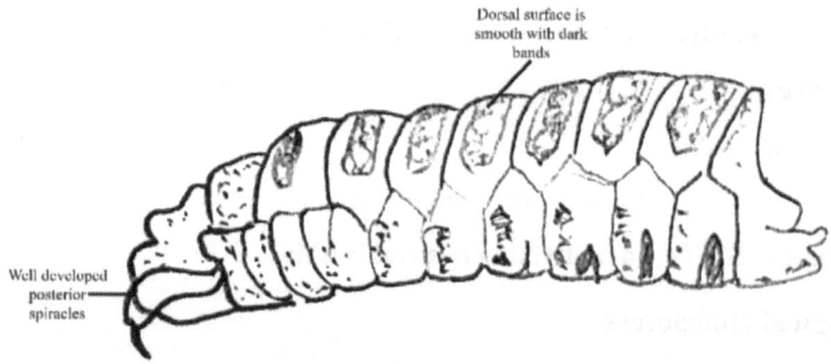

Figure 4.23. *Oestrus ovis* (Larva)

Life cycle: This fly itself is not parasitic but larvae are parasitic in upper respiratory tract. During fly season, fly goes on hovering around host. Occasionally, the flies drop on the body of animal particularly on head and larvae are deposited around nostrils. Larvae are very small, minute 1 mm long and pale yellow in colour. First stage larvae enter through nostrils into nasal passage or nasal chamber. In nasal chamber, they moult to 2nd stage larvae. L_2 continue migration deep into nasal chamber ultimately reaching the (cranial) frontal sinus. In frontal sinus, they moult to L_3.

Morphology of 3rd stage larvae: Narrow at anterior end and broad at posterior end. Body is made up of 12 segments. Anterior end is meant for attachment. Dorsal surface is convex while ventral surface is flat. **On dorsal side**, each segment has a **transverse dark band** while on ventral surface, each segment has 1 or 2 rows of spines. On last segment, there is pair of posterior spiracles. Each spiracular plate is D shaped with one central and many accessory openings. Third stage larvae (L_3) are found in frontal sinus of infected sheep around 35 days after infection. Larvae are thrown out by infected sheep with violent sneezing. On ground, these larvae penetrate into superficial layers of soil and moult to pupa. Pupal stage last for 3 to 6 weeks and then ultimately adult fly emerge out.

Habits

1. Fly attack animal in sheds or in pastures.
2. They prefer early morning sunlight.

Pathogenesis or Harmful effect

1. **Annoyance:** Adult flies hovering around host cause great annoyance. As a result, sheep try to run away from flies (Entomophobia). One particular tendency has been observed in sheep is that when flies attack them, they bunch together with their heads in center. This is done to prevent fly from depositing larvae in nostrils.
2. **Rhinitis/sinusitis:** Main pathogenesis is due to presence and development of larval stages in nasal chamber as well as in frontal sinus. So, during early phase of infection, there is rhinitis and watery discharge from nostrils. Later, discharge may become purulent due to secondary invasion by bacteria. Larvae which are present in sinus cause inflammation of sinus (sinusitis).
3. **Nervous signs:** Occasionally, L_3 may erode the skull bones and reach the CNS and cause damage or destruction of tissue of CNS and such sheep exhibit nervous symptoms like inclination of movement, circling and excitement. These types of symptoms are also seen in sheep suffering from "Gid" and hence this condition known as **"False Gid or pseudo-gid** ". To differentiate Gid from false Gid, there is no nasal discharge in case of gid but in false gid there is continuous mucopurulent discharge.

Diagnosis: Symptoms and at a time several sheep are infected with *Oestrus ovis*.

Treatment

1. Rafoxanide: @10mg/kg body wt. Orally, 100% efficacy.
2. Ivermectin: @ 0.2mg kg body wt. S/C route, 99.5% efficacy.
3. Closantel: @10mg/kg body wt. Orally, Two doses at 8 weeks interval. 98% effective.
4. Bromophos: 4% intranasal drops.
5. Dichlorovos: 3% intranasal spray.

Genus: *Hypoderma* (warble flies)

Species

Species	Common name	Hosts	Distribution
H. lineatum	Ox warble fly/cattle grub or heel fly	Cattle, deer rarely horse	Found in India
H. bovis	Ox warble fly/cattle grub	Cattle, deer rarely horse	European countries
H. crossi (Przhevalskiana silenus)	Goat warble fly	Goat and sheep	India

Morphological characters

1. These are medium size, 13 to 15 mm long and covered with coloured hair. Similarly veins of wings are also coloured.
2. On thorax, there are three silver lines and apex of abdomen bears orange-coloured hair.
3. Mouth part are rudimentary/vestigial.

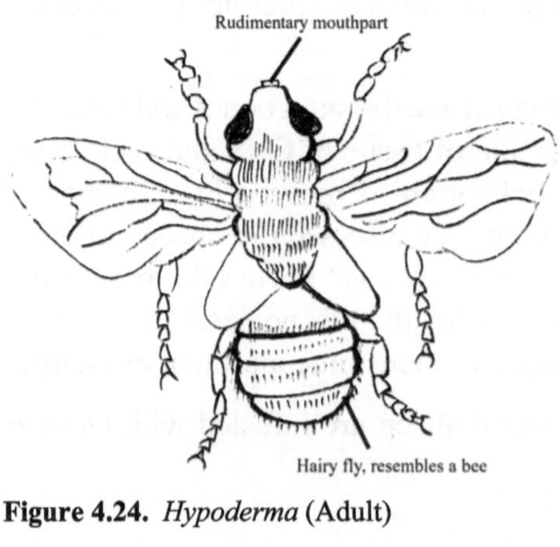

Figure 4.24. *Hypoderma* (Adult)

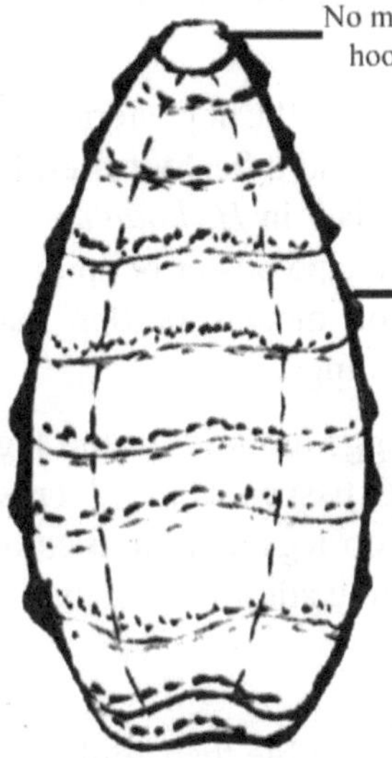

Figure 4.25. *Hypoderma* (Larva)

Life cycle of *H. bovis / H. lineatum*

They occur in month of May, June and July. Adults are not parasitic but larval stages are parasitic. Adult flies live for a very short period of 4 to 6 days, during this; they deposit 100 or more eggs on the body of the host. *Hypoderma bovis* lays one egg at a time on the single hair of rump or upper part of legs of cattle. *Hypoderma lineatum* lays 6 to 7 eggs at a time on single hair of legs or lower part of the body. *Hypoderma crossi* lays 6 to 7 eggs at a time. Eggs are 1 mm long and are attached to hair by small terminal clasps. Eggs hatch within 4 days and larva crawls down the hair and penetrates into skin to reach the subcutaneous tissue. They (L_1) wander in subcutaneous connective tissues and then towards diaphragm ultimately reaching **winter resting sites** which is **submucosal layer of oesophagus** for ***H. lineatum*** and **spinal canal or epidural fat** for ***H. bovis***. At these sites, larvae remain for 5 to 6 months and become second stage larvae (L_2). Second stage larvae then resume their migration and ultimately reach S/C tissue of back and migrate on either side of the vertebral column. Subsequently, L_2 form **swelling (warbles)** and make perforation in swelling. They remain here for 1-2 months **(spring resting sites)** keeping their posterior stigmal plates towards hole for breathing. After 8 days, they moult to L_3 and grow in size and as the size of larva increases, size of swelling also increases and these warbles become prominent. These L_3 remain inside warbles for one month and then subsequently wriggle out from warbles and drop on ground. Then they penetrate into superficial layer of soil and pupate. Pupal stage lasts for 35 days ultimately from pupa, adult come out. There is one cycle per year.

Morphology of L_3 larvae: L_3 is narrow at anterior end and flat at posterior end. It has 12 segments and, on each segment, there are around 8 **fleshy tubercles**. Small spines are also present in all segments except last in *H. linaetum* and last two in *H. bovis*. On last larval segments, kidney shape posterior spiracles are present which is pear shaped with deep notch on median border. Each spiracular plate has a central and many accessory openings.

***Hypoderma crossi*:** Usual host is sheep and goat. Eggs are laid on the legs. Egg hatch, L_1 come out, enters into skin to reach S/C tissues. L_1 of *H. crossi* does not migrate in S/C tissues. They form warbles on legs and larva comes out on to the ground to pupate and subsequently become adult.

Harmful Effects

Mostly cattle is affected. Young animals are more susceptible than adults.

1. **Entomophobia:** Adult flies are not parasitic but they go hovering around host for deposition of eggs so animal try to run away from flies and may get hurt. Entomophobia induce restlessness in animals causing disturbance in feeding and subsequent production loss. *Hypoderma* flies are active during day time and particularly attack animal standing in open sun.
2. **Main pathogenesis is due to tissue reaction to migrating larval stages.**
   i. **Oesophageal stenosis:** Tissue reaction to presence of large number of larvae in oesophageal wall cause stenosis of oesophageal lumen. This results in difficulty in swallowing.
   ii. **Paralysis:** Tissue reaction to larvae lodged in spinal canal and also damage caused by migrating larvae may result in paralysis of animals.
   iii. **Licked beef:** Along the route of migration, these larvae cause liquefaction of tissues or flesh along with greenish discoloration of flesh. Thus, heavily infected carcass has to be condemned. This liquefied flesh due to migration of larva of *Hypoderma* species also known as **"Butcher's jelly**." If butchers jelly is large in number, then whole carcass is condemned. If moderate in number, then carcass has to be trimmed i.e., removal of butcher's jelly and such carcass is known as "licked beef." This results in economic loss on accounts of carcass condemnation or trimming out of meat.

iv. **Secondary infections:** Warbles may become infected with bacteria and suppuration may take place. Similarly, these warbles make host susceptible for screw worm fly myiasis.

v. **Hide loss:** There is great loss to leather industry because of holes on skin and in heavily infested area, this amounts to lakhs of rupees.

Diagnosis

i. Warbles on skin.

ii. Presence of third stage larvae in warbles.

Treatment of *Hypoderma*

a. Old methods: Mechanical removal of larva from warbles with the help of forceps and if larva breaks inside the warbles, then there may be intense tissue reaction.

b. Ivermectin: @ 0.2mg/kg.b.wt. S/C

Order	:	**Diptera**
Suborder	:	Cyclorrhapha
Series	:	Schizophora
Section	:	Acalypterae

Character

1. Squammae small, not concealing halters.
2. Thorax without distinct transverse sutures.

Family: Gasterophilidae

Genus: *Gasterophilus*

Common name: 'Stomach bot' flies or 'horse bot' flies

Hosts: Horse and donkey

Type of disease: Gastric myiasis

General morphological characters of *Gasterophilus*

1. Large robust fly, about 1-2 cm in length.
2. Adult flies are brown in colour and hairy somewhat resembling bees.
3. Wings bear dark transverse bands across wing.
4. Mouthparts are reduced and functionless.

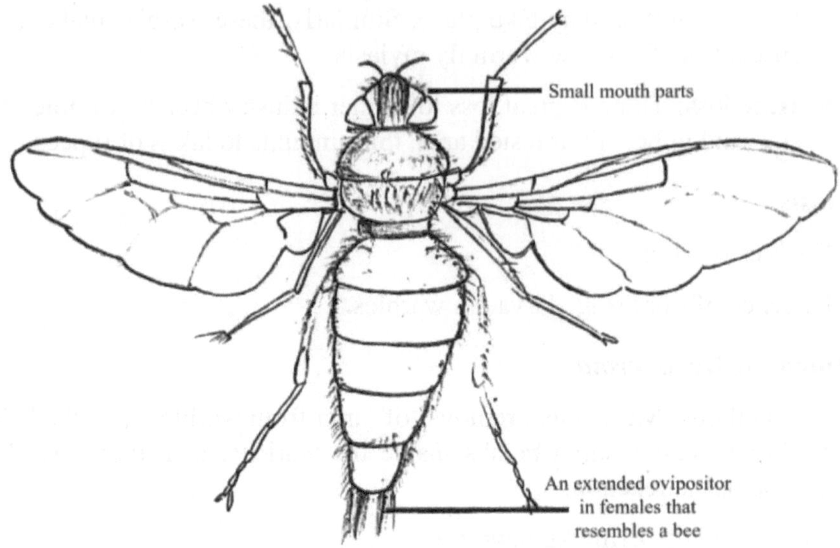

Figure 4.26. *Gasterophilus* (Adult)

Species: Different species are most readily recognized by the characters of third stage larvae.

Gasterophilus nasalis	:	Reported in India
G. intestinalis	:	Reported in India
G. pecorum	:	Reported in India
G. haemorrhoidalis	:	Not present in India
G. inermis	:	Not present in India

Life cycle: The flies are prevalent in summer season. Adult stage is not parasitic but larval stage are parasitic. Flies goes on hovering around horses with extended ovipositors and frequently drop down on body of host with extended ovipositors. Different species of *Gasterophilus* lay eggs at different places:

G. nasalis	:	Intermandibular region
G. intestinalis	:	Forelegs, particularly between scapula and fetlock
G. pecorum	:	Inanimate objects like saddle
G. haemorrhoidalis & *G. inermis*	:	Face particularly on cheeks

Eggs of *G. haemorrhoidalis* and *G. pecorum* are dark in colour and of other species are pale yellow. Eggs are pointed at attached end and operculate at the other. Eggs which are laid on head hatch spontaneously (4-10 days) and enter oral cavity through mouth or they penetrate through skin and enter oral cavity. Eggs of *G. intestinalis* & *G. pecorum* which are away from head are required to be licked for hatching and hatched larvae enter oral cavity while licking. First stage larvae instead of reaching stomach directly, they first penetrate mucosa of oral cavity, pharynx and tongue and wander here for several weeks, moult to second stage larvae and then L_2 stage comes in lumen of pharynx or oesophagus and reach the stomach. These L_2 stage attach gastric mucosa and become L_3.

(Larve of *G. intestinalis* attach cardiac portion of stomach rarely in fundus or pyloric and are reddish in colour. Larvae of *G. nasalis* are pale yellow and attach in the pylorus and the duodenum.

Larvae of *G. pecorum* are blood red in colour attach fundus region of stomach. Larvae of *G. haemorrhoidalis* any where in stomach and also in rectum when they pass out.)

Larvae remain in stomach for 10-12 months and mature L_3 is passed out along with the faeces, pupate on the ground and adult fly emerges in 3-5 weeks.

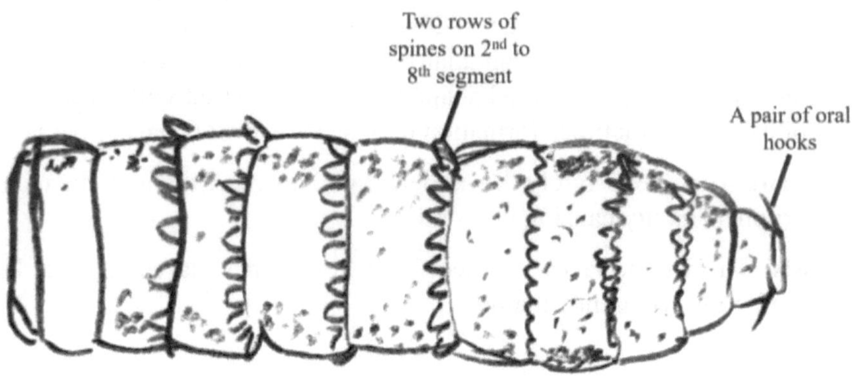

Figure 4.27. *Gasterophilus* (Larva)

Morphology of third stage larvae: Narrow at anterior end and broader at posterior end, 12 segmented each segment bears two rows of spines. **Spiracular plate is kidney shape and has three 'bow' shape slits.**

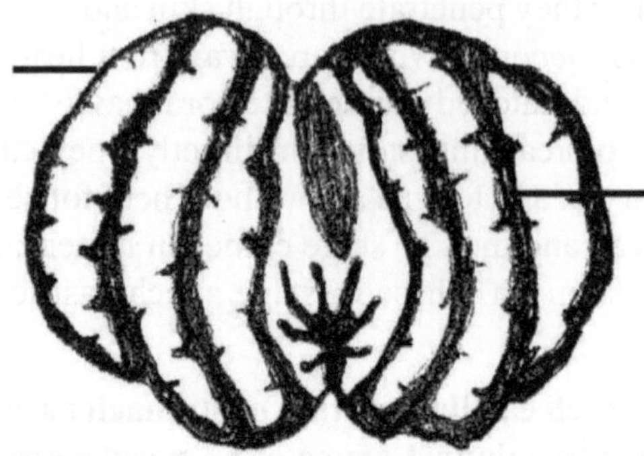
Semi-lunar shaped stigma plates
Three Semi-lunar shaped slits closely fused together in a pocket

Figure 4.28. Spiracle of *Gasterophilus* larva

Pathogenesis

1. **Entomophobia**
2. **Stomatitis**: Migration of larvae in oral mucosa cause stomatitis and infected horse show 'crib biting'. They also cause ulceration of tongue
3. **Gastritis** : Larvae which are present in mucosa cause catarrhal gastritis leading to formation of mucus. Digestion is not affected since larvae are usually attached to non-glandular part of stomach. In heavy infestation, there is formation of funnel shaped ulcer surrounded with hyperplastic epithelium. Sometimes formation of abscess occludes gastric passage.
4. **Peritonitis**: Very rarely larva penetrate gastric wall and then enter peritoneal cavity causing peritonitis.

Diagnosis: Third stage larvae in faeces. However, these larvae pass at later stage of infection when they mature.

Treatment

1. Carbon bisulphide: @ 10ml/50kg b.wt. through stomach tube or in gelatin capsule (old treatment).
2. Piperazine + Carbon bisulphide (Parvex) or Piperazine + Carbon bisulphide + Phenothiazine (Parvex plus) @ 110 mg/kg b.wt.
3. Trichlorophon: 39.6 mg/kg b. wt orally.
4. Dichlorovos: 26-53 mg/kg b. wt orally.
5. Inj. Ivermectin: 200-400 μg/kg b. wt S/C.

Control

1. Treatment of infected horses.
2. Frequent grooming. Horse should be sponged with water at 40-43°C to hatch larvae and water should contain insecticides to kill newly hatched larvae.

***Cobboldia elephantis*:** Elephant Bot Fly

The species found in stomach of elephant and also rhinoceros.

MYIASIS: word myiasis derived from greek word **'myia' which means fly.**

It is the infestation of animals or human with larvae of dipteran flies. Larvae feed on dead or living tissues. Myiasis can be classified on the basis of nature of fly and on the basis of organs infested:

Classification on the basis of nature of fly

1. **Obligatory myiasis:** Host is must for completion of life cycle. e.g. *Oestrus ovis*, *Gasterophilus* and *Hypoderma.*
2. **Facultative myiasis:** Myiasis caused by larvae of facultative myiasis where the host may or may not be required. e.g. *Calliphora, Lucilia, Sarcophaga* etc.
3. **Accidental myiasis:** Larvae of *Musca* developing in intestine of human being.

Classification on the basis organ infested

1. **Nasal myiasis:** *Oestrus ovis*
2. **Gastric myiasis:** *Gasterophilus*
3. **Somatic myiasis:** *Hypoderma*
4. **Cutaneous myiasis:** Calliphorid flies

Order	**:**	**Diptera**
Suborder	:	Cyclorrhapha
Series	:	Schizophora
Section	:	Pupipara

General characters

1. **Fly of this section are pupiparous**. Females lay fully matured larvae which pupate almost immediately.

2. Body is broad and flattened dorsoventrally.
3. Abdomen is mostly soft, leathery and indistinctly segmented.
4. **Legs ends in strong claws.**
5. Wings are present in some species and absent in others.
6. They are blood sucking flies.

Family: Hippoboscidae

1. Genus: *Hippobosca* (forest flies)

Species: *H. maculata* (Cattle), ***H. equina*** (Horse), ***H. longipennis*** (Dog)

Characters

1. Leathery, reddish brown with yellow spots on abdomen.
2. **Wing veins are crowded anteriorly.**

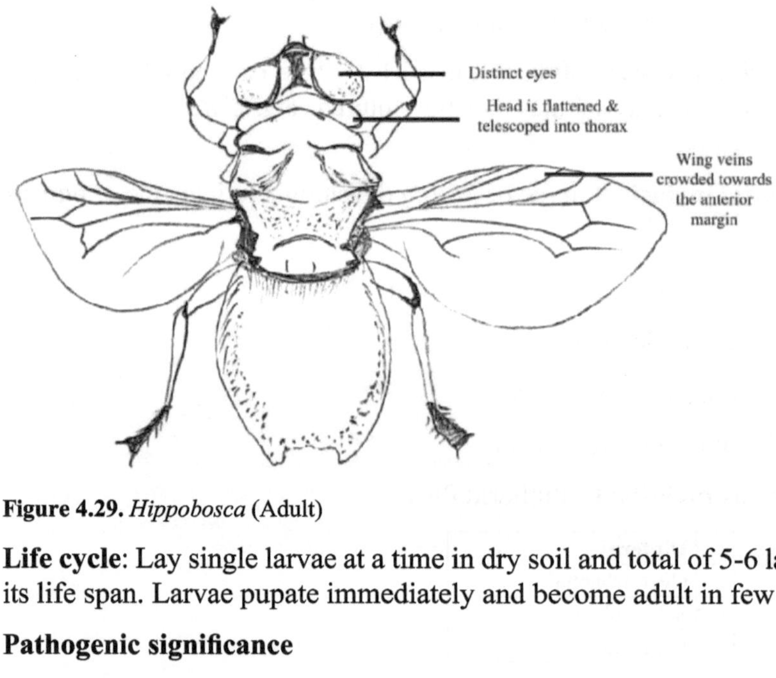

Figure 4.29. *Hippobosca* (Adult)

Life cycle: Lay single larvae at a time in dry soil and total of 5-6 larvae during its life span. Larvae pupate immediately and become adult in few days.

Pathogenic significance

1. Irritation to animals.
2. Vector: Transmit ***Trypanosoma theileri*** to cattle and ***Haemoproteus*** to birds.

2. Genus: *Melophagus*

Species: *Melophagus ovinus* (Sheep ked/tick fly/louse fly)

Host: Sheep

Distribution in India: In Kashmir region

Characters

1 They are **permanent ectoparasites and suck blood.**
2. **Head is short, broad and not freely movable.**
3. **Wingless insect.**
4. Transmission through **direct contact.**

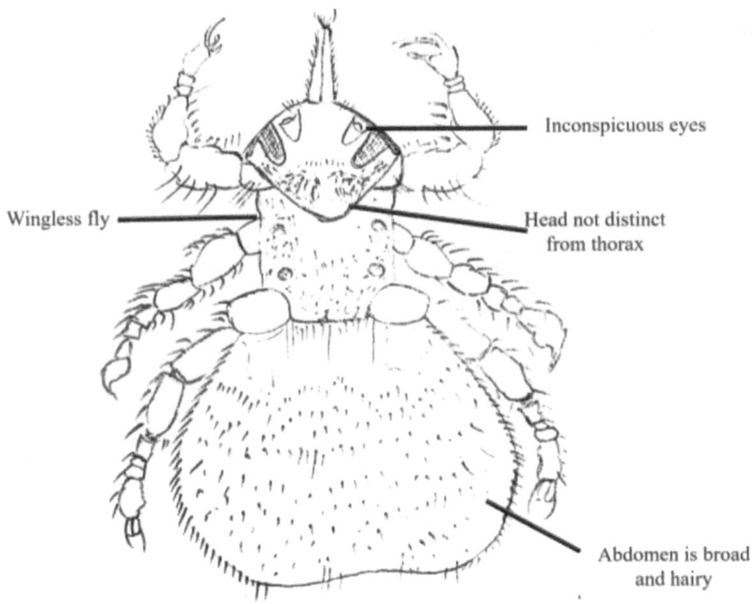

Figure 4.30. *Melophagus ovinus* (Adult)

Life cycle

Melophagus just like *Hippobosca*, lay single larva at a time but on the host and a total of 15 larvae are laid down by a female fly during its lifetime. Larvae is immobile and soon turns into a **chestnut brown pupa**. They also pupate immediately and adult emerges in 3-6 weeks depending upon the temperature.

The entire life is spent on the host and when off from the host, they die within 2-8 days.

Significance

(1) In heavy infection, cause anaemia.

(2) They cause intense irritation, as a result, sheep bite and rub themselves vigorously and damage the wool. **Faeces of ked stain the wool permanently thereby depreciating the economic value of the wool.**

(3) They act as a biological vector of ***Trypanosoma melophagium.***

3. Genus: *Pseudolynchia*

Species: *Pseudolynchia canariensis* (Bird fly/pigeon fly)

Host: Primarily pigeon and other birds

1. Blood sucking insects.
2. Tegument leathery.
3. Wings present.

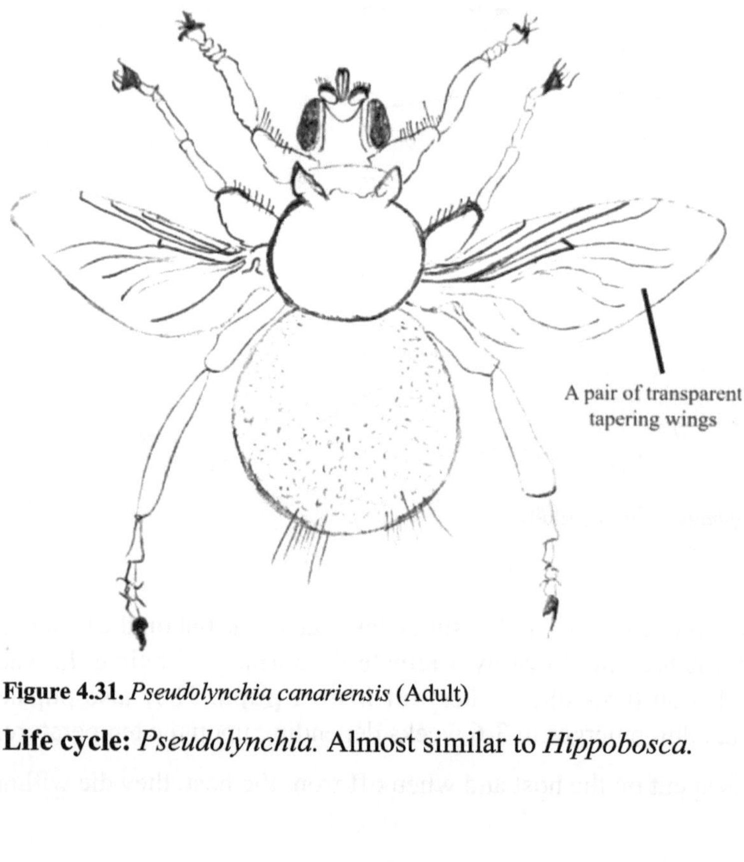

Figure 4.31. *Pseudolynchia canariensis* (Adult)

Life cycle: *Pseudolynchia.* Almost similar to *Hippobosca.*

Significance

(1) Biting is very painful to the bird.

(2) They suck blood and cause anaemia.

(3) Act as **biological vector of *Haemoproteus columbae.***

Control of Hippoboscid flies

(1) The best way is by spraying or dipping with insecticides.

(2) Regular shearing of wool can reduce the sheep ked population.

4. Genus: *Lipoptena*

Species: *Lipoptena caprina*

Host: Goat

Characters

1. **Both sexes of this genus have wings but cast when they find a host.**
2. The fly is leathery, brownish and head sunken into the thorax.

5

Order Coleoptera

Order: Coleoptera (beetles)

Class: Insecta

Subclass: Pterygota

Division: Endopterygota

Order: Coleoptera

Characters

1. They are commonly known as beetles.
2. It is the largest order and contributes 40% of total insects.
3. They bear two pairs of wings of which front pair is fully thickened, hence called as **elytra**, meet edge in the mid dorsal line act as hard or leathery cover for the posterior pairs of membranous wings.
4. Mouthparts are strongly mandibulated i.e. biting & chewing type.
5. Life cycle shows complete metamorphosis. Pupa is free or exarate type.

Pathogenic significance

1. Some beetles secrete a vesicating fluid when disturbed. This fluid contains a highly toxic agent, cantharadin. There is no immediate response but blister will be formed after 1-2 days.
2. Most of them act as crop pest.
3. Hair of some beetles may cause allergic reaction during inhalation.
4. Many of them act as intermediate hosts of different helminthes which are:

Tapeworms: *Raillietina cesticellus* (Poultry), *Choanotaenia infundibulm* (Poultry).

Round worms: *Spirocerca lupi* (oesophagus of dog), *Gongylonema pulchrum* (oesophagus of ruminants), stomach worms of pigs i.e. *Ascarops strongylina* and *Physocephalus sexalatus.*

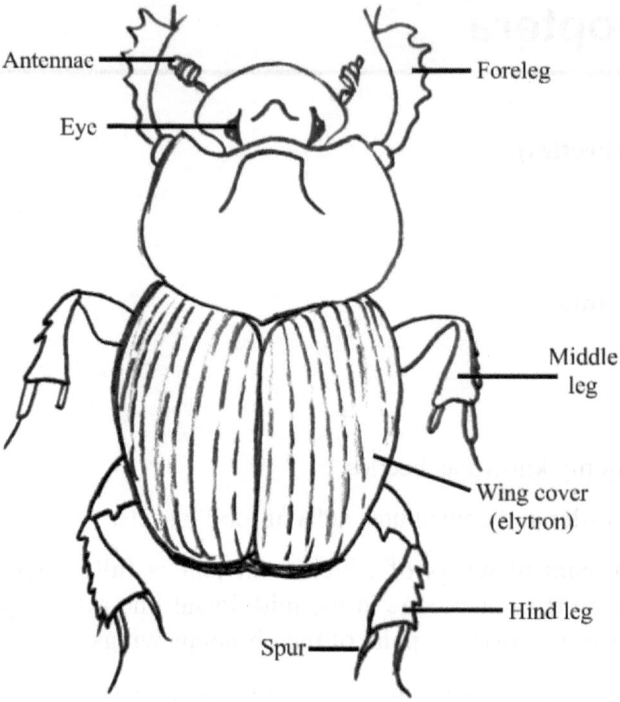

Figure 5.1. Coprophagus beetle

6

Order Siphonptera

Order: Siphonptera (Fleas)

Class: Insecta

Subclass: Pterygota

Division: Endopterygota

Order: Siphonaptera

Siphonaptera derived from two greek words viz. siphon (sucking) and apteron (wingless)

General characters of fleas

1. Body is laterally compressed.
2. Tegument is highly scleritized. Outer chitinous layer is very thick and it is dark brown in colour.
3. **A pair of simple eye or ocelli are present on head. Compound eyes absent.**
4. Short, clubbed antennae sunken in antennal groove.
5. Very small, wingless and 2 to 5mm long.
6. Mouth parts which are piercing and sucking type and are located along ventral margin of head.
7. Thorax made up of 3 segments. On each thoracic segment, there is a pair of very long legs. **Third pair is longest which helps the fleas in leaping.**
8. Abdomen made up of 10 segments and **on dorsal aspect of 9th segment**, there is a plate called **sensilium or pygidium** on which setae are present.
9. In some species, **"comb or ctenidia"** like structures are present. Comb present on ventral aspects of head called **"genal comb"** and those on posterior aspect of 1st thoracic segment called **''pronotal comb"**.
10. The **penis (aedeagus)** is chitinous and coiled.

Different species of fleas

Species of fleas	Common name	Host	Characters
Ctenocephalides canis	Dog flea	Dog	Genal and pronotal comb or ctenidia present. First spine of genal comb is smaller than rest. Head is square in shape.
Ctenocephalides felis	Cat flea	Cat	Genal and pronotal comb present. All spines of genal comb are equal. Head is elongated.
Echidnophaga gallinacea	Stick tight flea	Birds	Genal and pronotal comb absent. Head is angulate.
Pulex irritans	Human flea	Human	Comb or ctenidia absent. Presence of ocular seta or spine below eye.
Xenopsylla cheopis	Oriental or black rat flea	Rat	Comb or ctenidia absent. Presence of ocular seta or spine in front of eye.
Ceratophyllus gallinae	Common flea of chicken	Bird	Only pronotal comb present.
Tunga penetrans	Jigger/ Chigoe	Man and pig	Frons sharply angled.

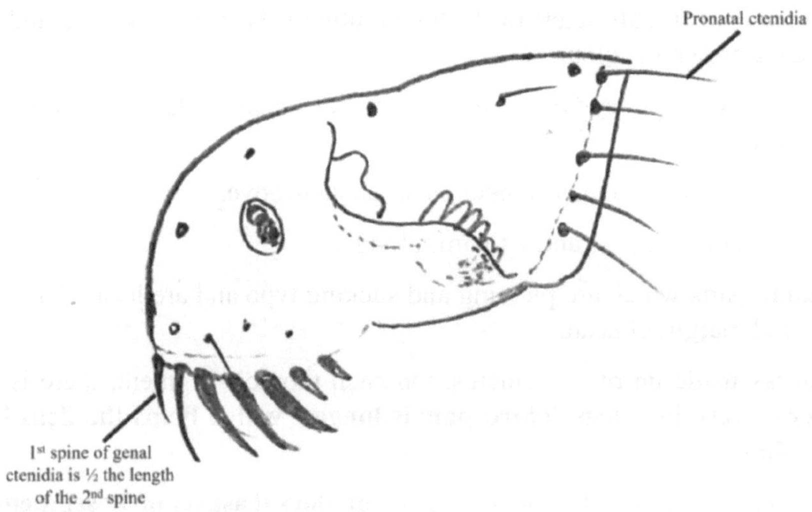

Figure 6.1. *Ctenocephalides canis* (Head)

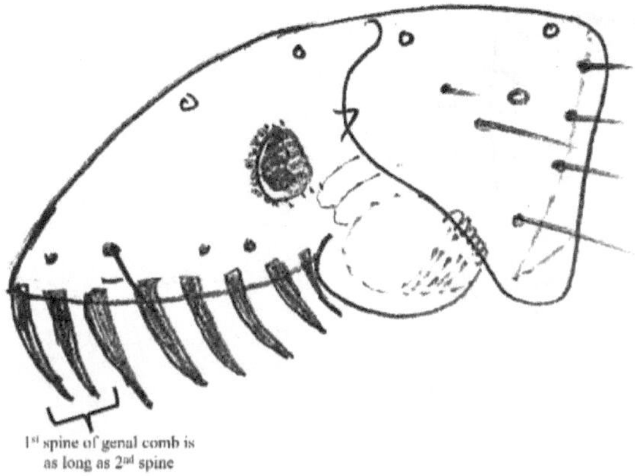

Figure 6.2. *Ctenocephalides felis* (Head)

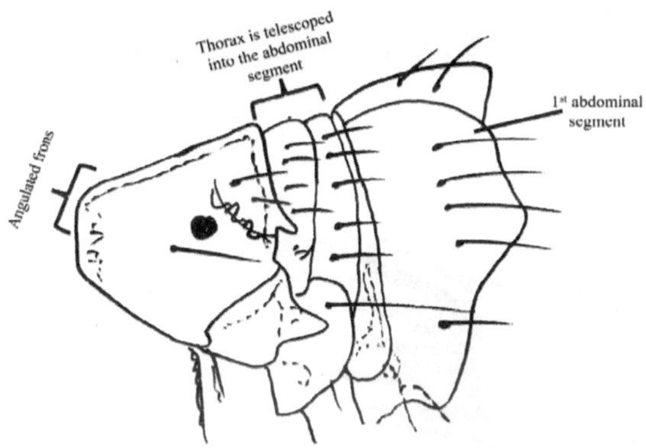

Figure 6.3. *Echidnophaga gallinacea* (Head)

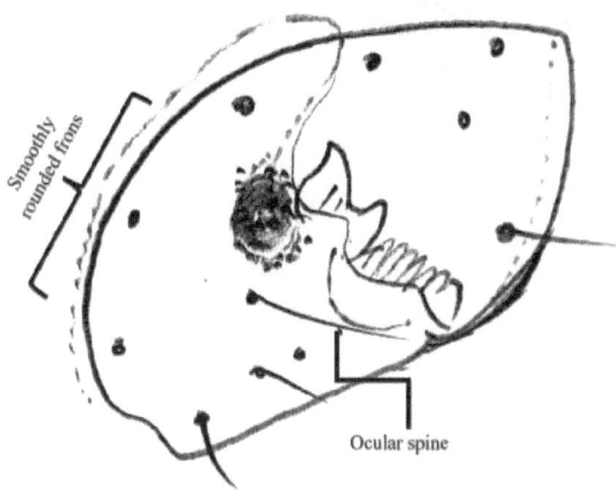

Figure 6.4. *Pulex irritans* (Head)

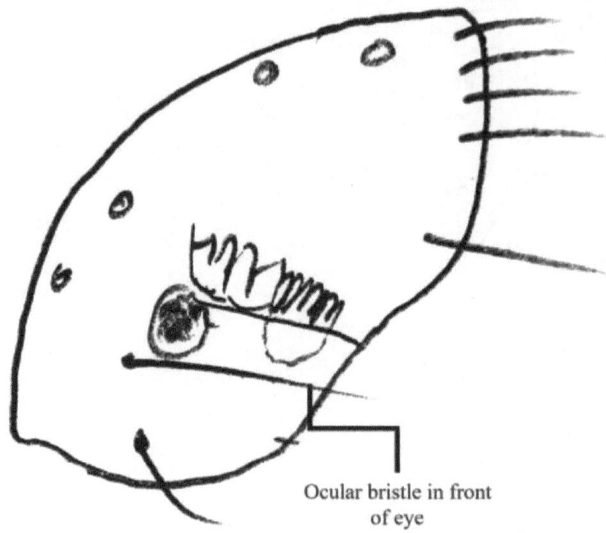

Figure 6.5. *Xenopsylla cheopis* (Head)

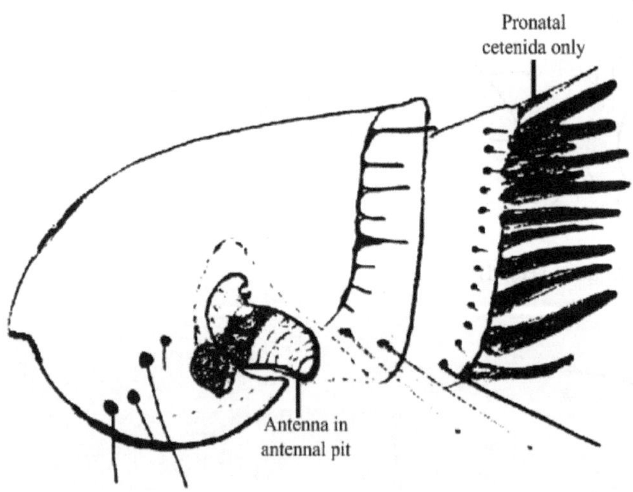

Figure 6.6. *Ceratophyllus gallinae* (Head)

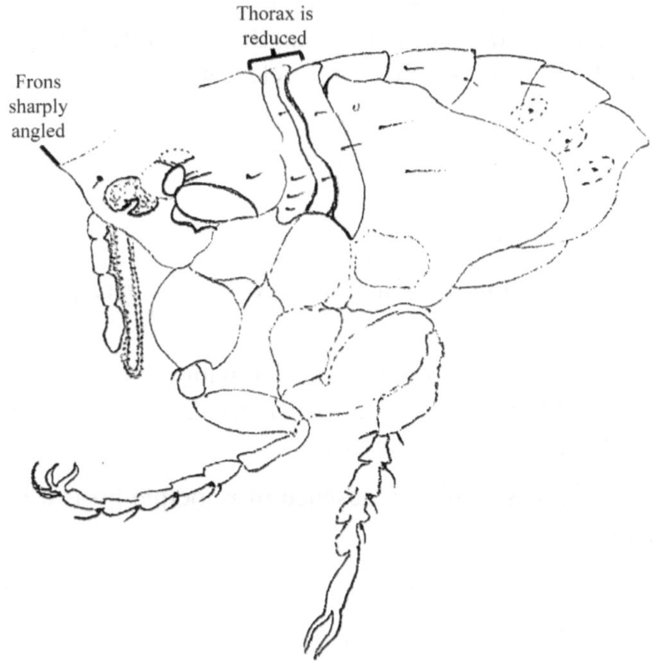

Figure 6.7. *Tunga penetrans*

Life cycle of fleas in general

The female fleas lay around 20 eggs at a time and 300-400 eggs during its life span. Eggs are deposited on the dirt and dust material at the corner of animal and poultry houses. Occasionally egg is laid on body of host usually such eggs drop down immediately. Egg is small, 0.5 mm in length, whitish in color with rounded ends. Development of larva inside eggs depends on suitable climatic condition. Eggs hatch within 2-16 days and larva comes out. Larvae are elongated, slender and maggot like. Larva is whitish in colour and body consists of small head at anterior end, 3 thoracic segments and 10 abdominal segments. On head, there is chitiouns spine with the help of which larva breaks shell of eggs and come out. **Masticatory type mouth part with which larvae feed upon dry faeces and organic matter**. Entire larval body is covered with hair. On last larval segment, there is a pair of stiff spines and these spines are called as **"anal struts"** which are meant for locomotion. In corner of animal house, they survive for 7 to 10 days at the end of which, **larva spins a cocoon around itself and inside cocoon it moults to pupa.** Pupa stage is passed inside cocoon and it lasts 10 to 11 days, at the end of which, adult flea comes out. **In case of *Echidnophaga gallinacea,* flea burrow deep inside skin**

forming nodules and ulcers and, in these nodules, eggs are laid. Then these eggs hatch on body of the host and larvae comes out. Subsequently, the larvae drop down from the host body and rest of the life cycle is same.

Habits of fleas

1. **Suck blood.**
2. They are **temporary parasites.**
3. They move by **jumping action** called hopping and the protein responsible is **resilin.**
4. Longevity of adult stages depends upon climatic conditions i.e. temperature and humidity that affect feeding pattern. Unfed fleas cannot survive for longer time during dry conditions.
5. Fleas are not rigidly host specific, in absence of principle host, it may attack another animal also.

Significance

1. **Anaemia:** Fleas are blood sucker, so in heavily infested host, they may lead to anaemia.
2. **Hypersensitivity reaction:** Bites of fleas are painful, irritating and saliva of flea is allergic so during initial exposure, host is sensitized to saliva of flea and when this sensitized host is again exposed to flea, then there is severe hypersensitive reaction. As a result, area becomes red due to formation of papules which may lead to pustules formation as a result of bacterial invasion and urticarial patches. This condition is known as "**Flea bite dermatitis**".

   In **cats**, this condition is more severe resulting into reddish focal spots on the skin and condition in cat is also known as "**Milliary dermatitis**".
3. **Vector:** Flea also acts as intermediate host like:
   - ***Ctenocephalides canis* and *C. felis* for *Dipylidium caninum* and also for *Dipetalonema reconditum***
   - ***Xenopsylla cheopis* transmits Bubonic plague** caused by *Pasteurella* or *Yersinia pestis*.
   - Rat flea also transmit *Trypanosoma lewisi*, Tularaemia (*Pasteurella tulariensis*) and murine typhus (*Rickettsia mooseri*)
4. The stick tight flea, *Echidnophaga gallinacea* attacks poultry and other birds and are found in clusters on comb, wattle and eyes of birds causing

itching, emaciation, anaemia, nodules, ulcers, drop in production and mortality in heavy infection.

Control

1. Treatment of affected birds: spray or dusting of birds with suitable insecticides like Chlorolane or Methoxychlor @ 5% powder for dusting and 0.5% as spray.
2. Lindane @ 0.1% for dusting and 0.06% as spray.
3. Organophosphorous compound like Malathion and Sumithion @ 0.05-0.14% for application on body.
4. Pyrethroides compound are also effective and safe like deltamethrin, Butox etc.
5. Certain herbal preparation like Pestoban has to be diluted 10 times before use.
6. Dog soaps, shampoo containing Tetmosole.
7. **Flea collars** are available. Flea collrs made of polyvinyl chloride and impregnated with dichlorovos.

   Flea collar for dog: 9.3% of dichlorovos.

   Flea collar for cat: 4.65% of dichlorovos.

   This gives protection for 3-6 months. Once collar is applied, use of any other organophosphorous compound on the body is prohibited.
8. For treating bird for stick tight flea, DDT or Chlorolane or Methoxychlor @1% for dusting and 0.1% for spray is suitable.
9. **Insect development inhibitor (IDI) like lufeneuron** can be used orally to inhibit chitin synthesis and eggs and larval development.

7

Order Mallophaga and Siphunculata

Lice

Class: Insecta

Subclass: Pterygota

Division: Exopterygota

Order: Mallophaga (Biting louse) and order Siphunculata or Anoplura (sucking louse)

General characters of lice

1. **Lice are permanent obligatory ecto-parasites** of animals and birds.
2. They are **very host and site specific.**
3. Lice are dorsoventrally flattened, **wingless creatures.**
4. Body is divided into head, thorax and abdomen.
5. Eyes are reduced or absent in certain species. Compound eyes are absent.
6. Antennae are short.
7. Thorax is made up 3 segments however, the segmentation is indistinct. Each segment is having one pair of stumpy legs and at end of which one or two claws are present. One pair of spiracles present on mesothorax.
8. **Metamorphosis is incomplete type**

Difference between biting and sucking louse

	Siphunculata (Sucking Louse)	Mallophaga (Biting Louse)
1.	Head is conical anteriorly.	Head is rounded or flattened anteriorly.
2.	Sucking lice.	Biting lice.
3.	Mouth parts are adopted for piercing and sucking action.	Mouth parts are adopted for biting action.
4.	Thoracic segmentation is indistinct.	Prothorax is prominent. Meso and meta thoracic segment fused to form pterothorax.
5.	Spiracle on thorax is on dorsal side.	Spiracle on thorax is on ventral side.
6.	Parasitic only on mammalian host.	Parasitic on mammalian as well as on avian host.

Order: Mallophaga

Characters: 1. Eyes are vestigial.

2. Tarsus bears two claws in bird lice and one claw in mammal lice.

Three suborders: Amblycera, Ischnocera and Rhynchophthirina

Difference between Amblycera and Ischnocera:

Amblycera	Ischnocera
Antennae arise from antennal groove.	Antennae arise from lateral margin of head and antennal groove is absent.
Third antennal segment is stalked.	No such stalk.
Maxillary palps are present.	Maxillary pulps are absent.
Nine abdominal segments.	Eight abdominal segments.

Sub-order Amblycera

Avian lice

a. *Menopon gallinae*: **Shaft louse of poultry**

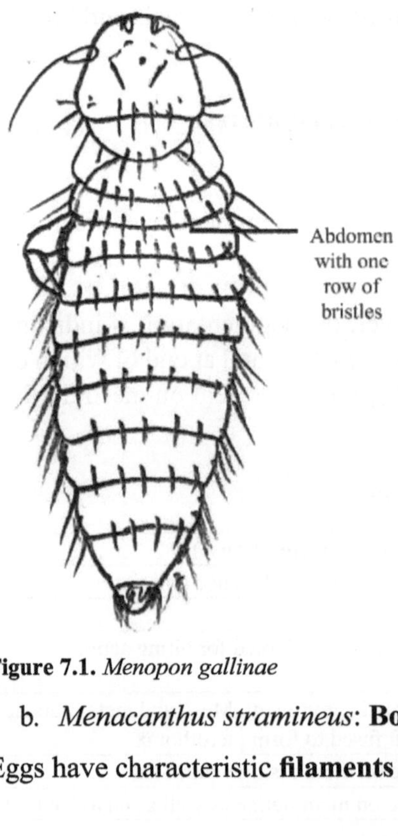

Figure 7.1. *Menopon gallinae*

b. *Menacanthus stramineus*: **Body louse of poultry**.

Eggs have characteristic **filaments on anterior half of eggs.**

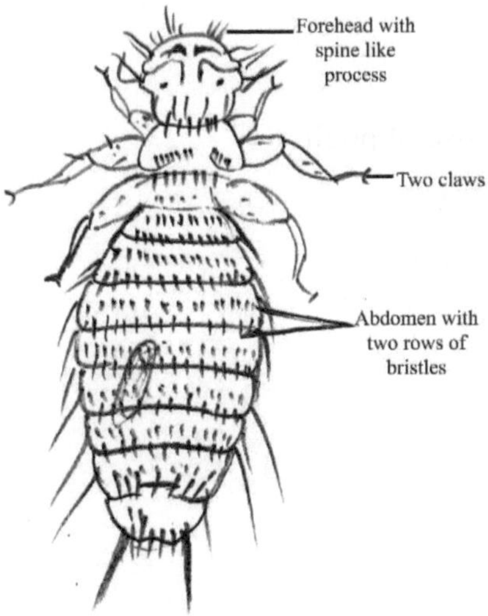

Figure 7.2. *Menacanthus stramineus*

c. *Trinoton anserinum*: Ducks

d. *Holomenopon leucoxanthum* (cause of **wet feather of ducks)**

Mammalian lice

Genus: *Heterodoxus*

Heterodoxus spiniger: common on dogs in India. **This louse has two claws per legs and is an exception amomg mammalian louse.**

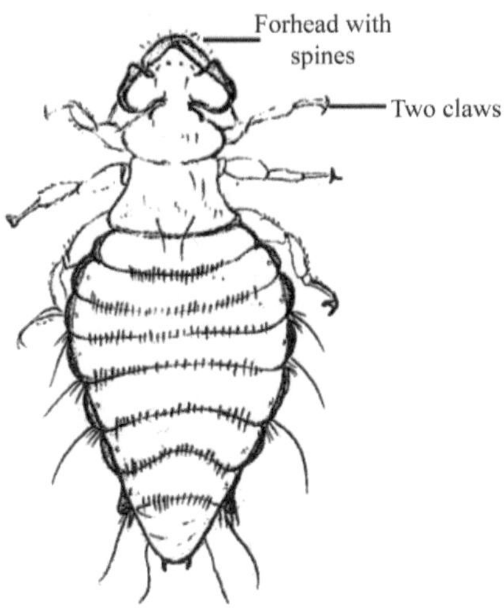

Figure 7.3. *Heterodoxus spiniger*

Sub-order Ischnocera

Avian lice

1. ***Cuclotogaster heterogaphus*: Head louse of poultry**
2. ***Lipeurus caponis*: Wing louse of poultry**
3. ***Goniocotes gallinae*: Fluff louse of poultry**
4. ***Gonoides gigas*: Large louse of poultry**
5. ***Columbicola columbae*: (Pigeons)**
6. ***Anaticola anseris*: (Duck)**

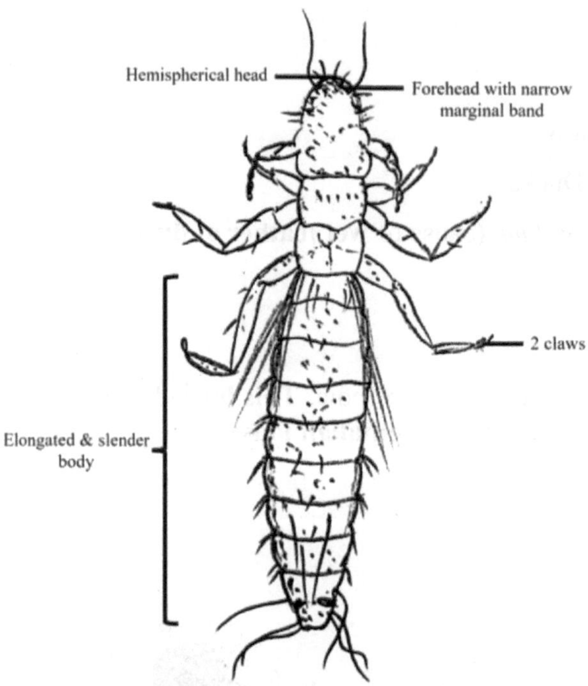

Figure 7.4. *Lipeurus caponis*

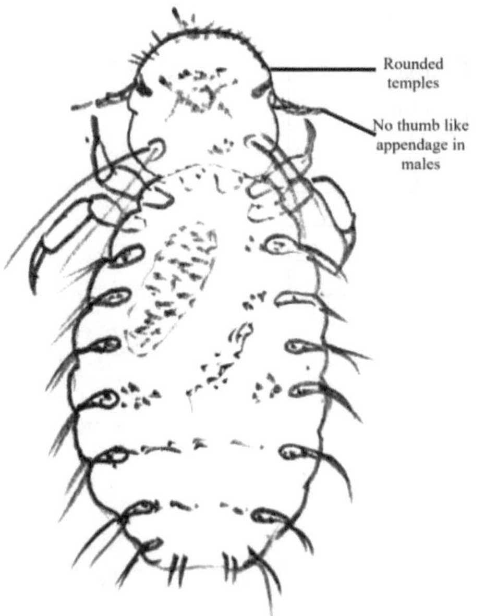

Figure 7.5. *Goniocotes galilnae*

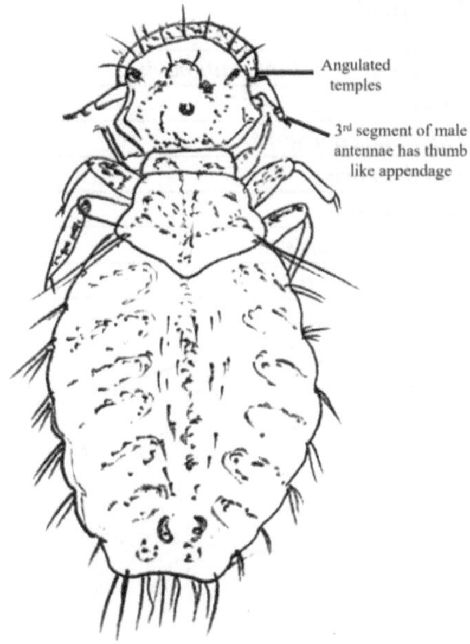

Figure 7.6. *Gonoides gigas*

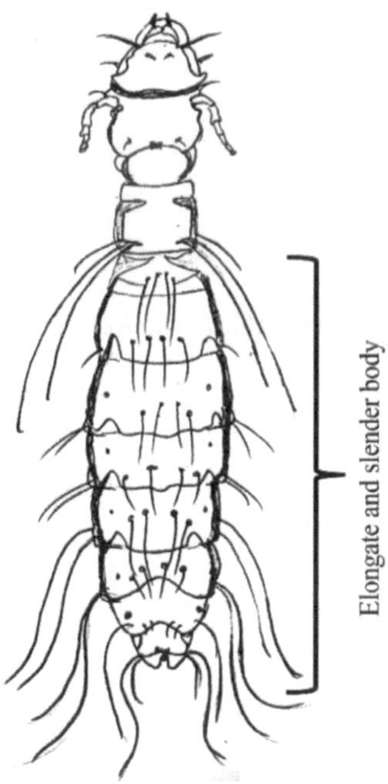

Figure 7.7. *Columbicola columbae*

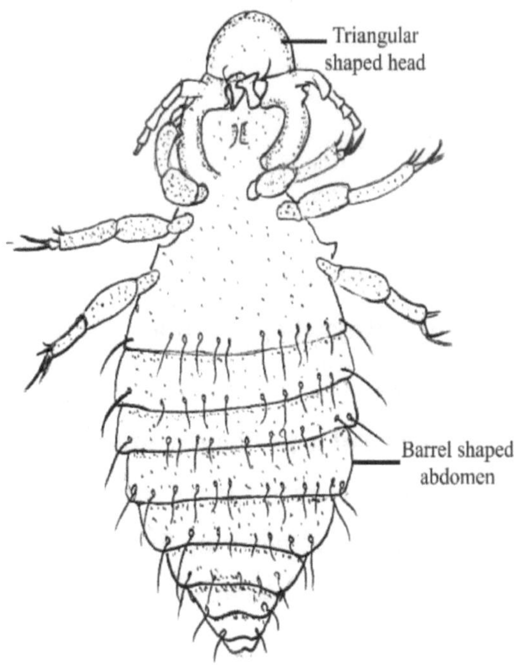

Figure 7.8. *Cuclotogaster heterogaphus*

Mammalian lice

Damalinia (syn. Bovicola) bovis	Cattle
Damalinia equi	Equine
Damalinia caprae	Goat
Damalina ovis	Sheep
Damalina suis	Swine
Trichodectis canis	Dog
Felicola subrostratus	Cat

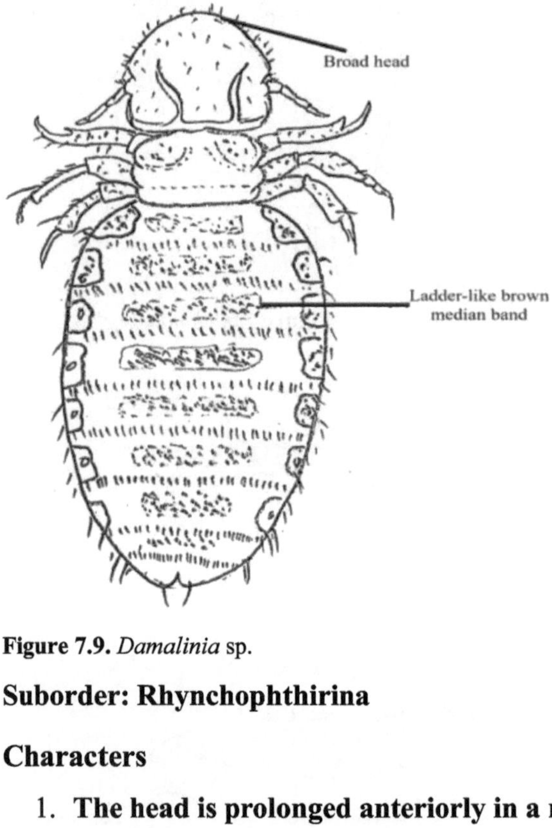

Figure 7.9. *Damalinia* sp.

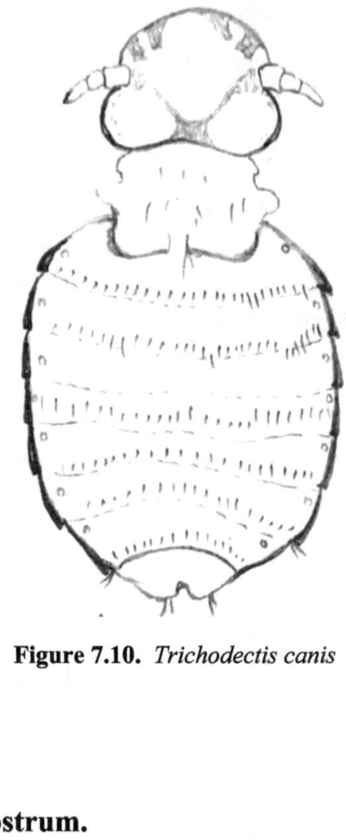

Figure 7.10. *Trichodectis canis*

Suborder: Rhynchophthirina

Characters

1. **The head is prolonged anteriorly in a rostrum.**
2. Mandible are at apex of rostrum.
3. Thoracic segments are fused.

***Haematomyzus elephantis*:** Occurs on Indian and African elephant

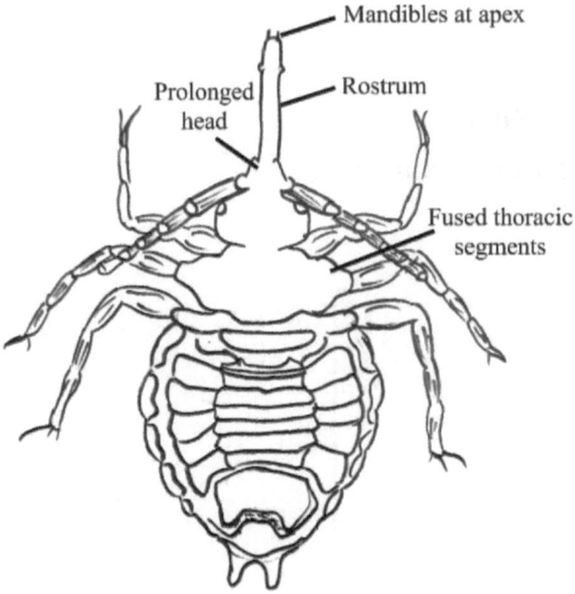

Figure 7.11. *Haematomyzus elephantis*

Order: Anoplura or Siphunculata

Characters

1. **Sucking lice. Mouth Parts adapted for piercing the skin.**
2. Parasites of mammals only.
3. Head is prolonged anteriorly.
4. Tarsus bears one prominent claw and a tibial pad.

Family: Haematopinidae

Characters

1. Eyes are absent.
2. Head has forward prolongations **(temporal angles)** behind the antennae.
3. Thorax is broad and has **marked paratergal plates.**
4. One row of spines on each abdominal segment.

Genus: *Haematopinus*

Species

Haematopinus tuberculatus **(buffalo)**

Haematopinus eurysternus **(short nose cattle louse)**

Haematopinus suis **(pig)**

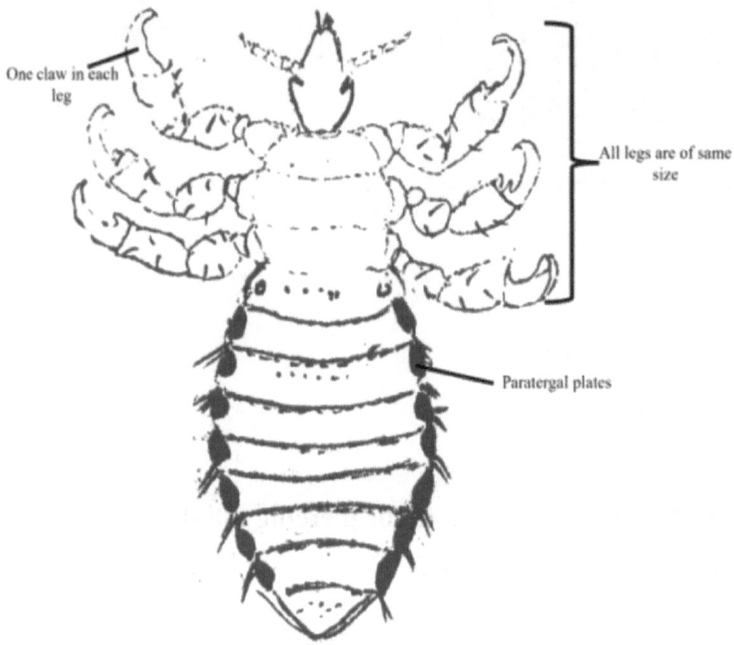

Figure 7.12. *Haematopinus eurysternus*

Family: Linognathidae

Characters

1. Eyes are absent.
2. Abdomen is membranous with numerous hair on segments.
3. The first pair of legs are smallest.

Genus: *Linognathus*

Linognathus ovillus: Blue louse of sheep/ face louse/body louse of sheep

Linognathus vituli: Long nosed louse of cattle

Linognathus pedalis: **Foot louse of sheep**

Linognathus setosus: **dog and foxes**

Linognathus stenopis: **goats**

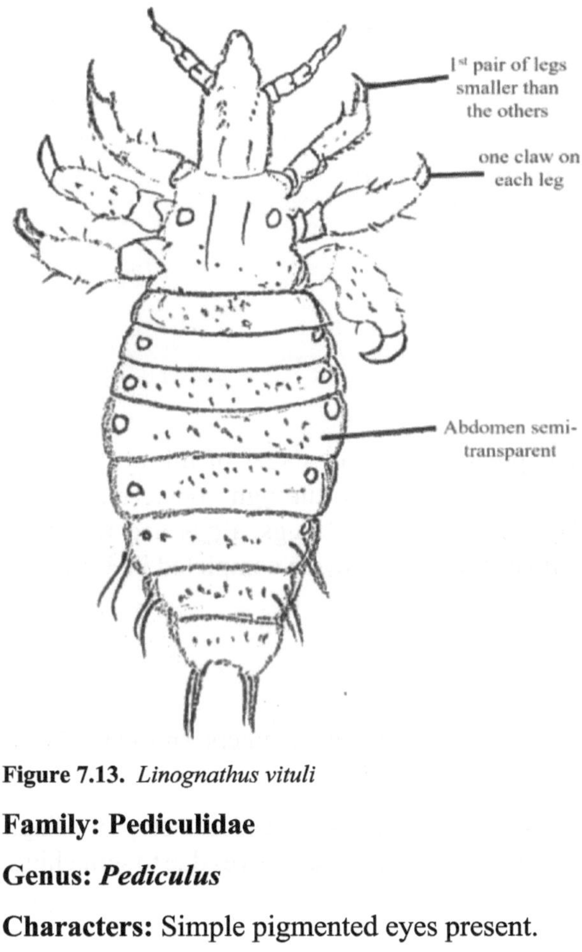

Figure 7.13. *Linognathus vituli*

Family: Pediculidae

Genus: *Pediculus*

Characters: Simple pigmented eyes present.

Species: *Pediculus humanus:* Human head louse

Phthirus pubis: Human pubic louse/crab louse

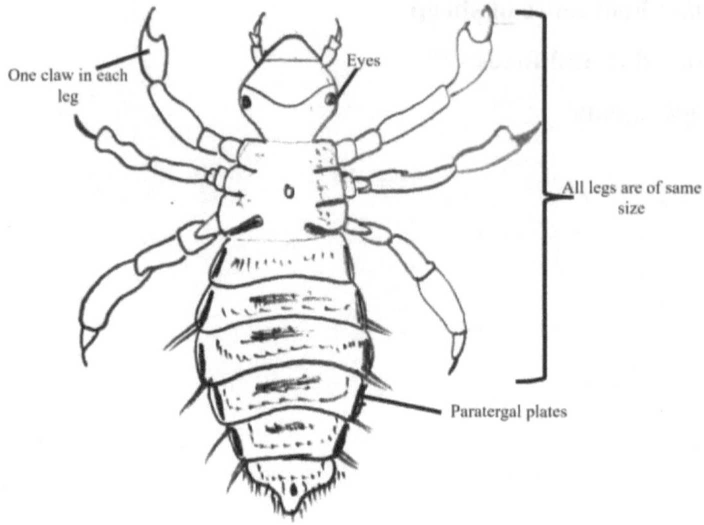

Figure 7.14. *Pediculus sp.*

Life cycle: Lice are permanent parasites and all stages of life cycle occur on body of same host. Transmission takes place through contact and farm equipments. A female louse lays around 200-300 eggs. **Eggs are white in colour, operculated and are called "nits".** Life cycle completed in 3 weeks.

Significance

Birds

1. Avian lice feed on dermal scales, scabs and feathers and can **digest keratin.**
2. They cause irritation, itching, birds become restless, stop feeding, anaemia and drop in production. They injure themselves due to scratching and feather plucking.

Mammals

1. Irritation, scratching, injury, loss of hair, wounds and damage of hide particularly by biting louse.
2. Loss of wool in sheep that may result in myiasis.
3. Frequent licking of itching region may result in ingestion of hair and subsequently formation of hair balls in stomach leading to digestive disturbances.

4. Act as Intermediate host: *Trichodectes canis* for dog tape worm (*Dipylidium caninum*).

Control and Treatment: Similar to fleas.

Difference between Flea and Louse

Flea	Louse
Laterally compressed.	Dorsoventrally compressed.
Life cycle stages are egg, larva, pupa and adult.	Life cycle stages are egg, larva, nymph and adult.
Fleas are temporary parasites.	Louse is permanent parasites.
Legs are every long.	Legs are short.
Fleas are not rigidly host specific.	Not only host but also region specific.

8

Order Hemiptera

Bugs

Class: Insecta

Subclass: Pterygota

Division: Exopterygota

Order: Hemiptera (Bugs)

Characters

1. These are true bugs.
2. Mouth parts adapted for piercing and sucking. Proboscis kept folded in head when not in use.
3. Two pairs of wings usually present, anterior harder pair called **hemelytra**. Posterior pair is membranous.
4. Both male and female are blood suckers.
5. Metamorphosis is incomplete.

Family: Cimicidae

Genus: *Cimex lectularius*

Characters

1. Commonly called **bed bugs**.
2. They are 4-5 mm long, flat bodied, elongate oval in shape and yellowish-brown to dark brown in colour.
3. A pair of long antennae with four joints.
4. Compound eyes project conspicuously at the sides of head.
5. The prothorax is deeply notched where head is inserted.
6. Wings are vestigial.

7. Adult has a pair of ventral thoracic stink glands. In young stage have similar dorsal abdominal glands. These stink glands are responsible for typical odour of bed bug.

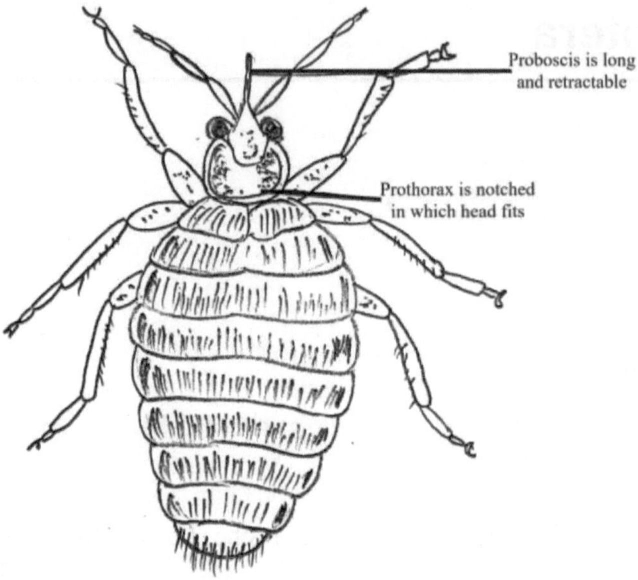

Figure 8.1. *Cimex lectularius*

Life cycle: The adult female lays eggs in cracks and crevices which then give rise to larvae which further undergo incomplete metamorphosis to form five nymph stages followed by adult.

Significance: They are nocturnal in habits, voracious blood sucker. Biting is painless during feeding but becomes painful later. They do not transmit any disease.

Family: Reduvidae

Genus: *Triatoma*

Common name: Reduvid bug/Kissing bug/Assassin bug/Cone-nose shaped bug (prefers to bite on cheek)

Character

1. Head is elongated and cone shaped.
2. Nocturnal.
3. Biting painless.

Significance: They transmit *Trypanosoma cruzi*. This bug is not present in India.

Control: As for fleas and lice.

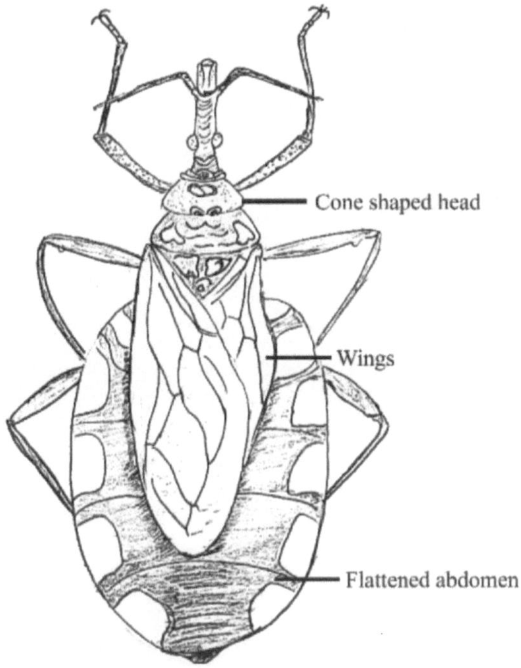

Figure 8.2. *Triatoma*

9

Order Orthoptera and Odonata

Order: Orthoptera

This order includes **cockroaches and grasshoppers**. They bear the following characters:

1. The body is oval and flattened in cockroach and elongated in grasshopper.
2. Two pairs of wings are present. Mesothoracic pair of wings is thickened **(Tegmina)** and act as cover for membranous metathoracic pair of wings.
3. Antennae are long and multi-jointed.
4. The legs are modified for fast running (cockroach) or jumping (grasshopper).
5. Metamorphosis is incomplete.

Importance

They act as vector or intermediate host of different parasites.

Cockroach

(i) *Gongylonema pulchrum* (Oesophageal worm of ruminants and pig)

(ii) *Oxyspirura mansoni* (Eye worm of poultry)

(iii) *Physaloptera praeputialis* (Stomach worm of cat)

Grasshopper

(i) *Tetrameres americana* and *T. mohtedai* (Proventricular worm of poultry)

(ii) *Cheilospirura hamulosa* (Gizzard worm of poultry)

(iii) *Physaloptera praeputialis* (Cat)

(iv) *Eurytrema pancreaticum* (Ruminants duct flukes).

(v) *Choanotaenia infundibulum* (Poultry tape worm).

Order: Odonata

1. They are **dragon fly.**
2. They are predator insects.
3. Presence of large eyes and antennae are hair like.
4. Mouth parts chewing type.
5. Metamorphosis is incomplete.
6. Eggs are laid in water; nymph is aquatic and are called **naiad.**

Significance: Naiads act as second intermediate host for oviduct fluke i.e. *Prosthogonimus* spp.

10

Important Characters and Classification of Class Arachnida

Class- Arachnida

- Class Arachnida includes scorpions, spiders, ticks and mites.
- Antennae, wings and compound eyes are absent.
- Body divided into head, thorax and abdomen.
- Mouth is small and adapted for suck blood or tissue fluids of host.
- Most of the members have poison glands or claws for paralyzing the host before sucking.
- The first and second pair of appendages is known as chelicerae and pedipalps, respectively.
- The first six segments of body are termed as prosoma and rest segments as opisthosoma.
- The prosoma bears appendages containing chelicerae and pedipalps, jointly known as gnathosoma and four pairs of walking legs known as podosoma.

Chelicerae	=	1st pair of appendages
Pedipalps	=	2nd pair of appendages
Prosoma	=	1st six segments of body
Opisthosoma	=	Segments of body except prosoma
Gnathosoma	=	Bears appendages (chelicerae and pedipalps)
Podosoma	=	Bears four pairs of walking legs
Opisthosoma	=	Bears abdomen
Idiosoma	=	Podosoma+ Opisthosoma

- In case of ticks and mites, external signs of segmentation are not evident thus, body is divided into two parts-

  a. **Gnathosoma or capitulum** (anterior portion, bearing chelicerae, pedipalps and a median hypostome). These are mouth parts of ticks and mites modified for holding on body of host and sucking blood.

  b. **Idiosoma** (posterior portion made by fusion of podosoma and opisthosoma).

- Respiration takes place by means of gill-books (in aquatic species), lung-books and tracheae (in terrestrial species) or general body surface (species in which specialized organs for respiration are absent).

The basic difference between Insecta and Arachnida are-

Character	Insecta	Arachnida
Body	Body is divided into head, thorax and abdomen.	Head and thorax are fused, body is divided into cephalothorx and abdomen.
Antennae	Present.	Absent.
Mouthparts	Consists of a labrum, labium, hypopharynx, mandibles (1 pair) and maxillae (1 pair).	Comprises of paired chelicerae, paired palps and central hypostomes.
Eyes	Compound eyes usually present, simple eye present in some species.	Compound eyes absent. Simple eye present.
Legs	Adult have three pairs of leg.	Adult have four pairs of leg.
Wings	Present or absent.	Absent.
Excretory organ	Malphigian tubules.	Malphigian tubules and coxal glands (true nephridia).
Life cycle	Holometabolous (complete) or Hemimetabolus (incomplete).	Hemimetabolus (incomplete).

Classification of arachnids

Kingdom : Animalia
Phylum : Arthropoda
Sub-phylum : Chelicerata
Class : Arachnida
Sub-class : Acari (Acarina)
Order: Parasitiformes, Acariformes

Sub-order: Ixodida, Gamasida, Actiniedida, Acaridida and Oribatida

Example: Ticks and Gamsid mites

General characters of Sub-class Acarina

1. Acarina includes **ticks (macroscopic)** and **mites (microscopic)**.
2. Segmentation on body is indistinct i.e. no external signs of segmentation.
3. Body is divided into **gnathosoma or capitulum** (bears chelicerae, pedipalps and median hypostome) and idiosoma (comprises of podosoma bearing four pairs of legs and opisthosoma which correspond to abdomen).
4. Chelicerae is saw like structure used for cutting the tissues, palp has sensory function and a hypostome consists of rows of recurved teeth and has dorsal groove for passage of blood, saliva etc.
5. In addition to palps, there is another sensory structure called **Haller's organ** present on the **last segment of first pair of legs**.
6. Respiration is performed by tracheal system in ticks while parasitic mites respire through cuticle.
7. They have incomplete or hemimetabolus type of life cycle and includes-

   Egg ⟶ Larva ⟶ Nymph ⟶ Adult
8. **Larva have only 3 pairs of legs** (4th pair of legs are absent).
9. Nymphs resembles with adult stage except presence of genital organs. One or more nymphal stages called protonymph, deutonymph and tritonymph may be present in lifecycle.

Difference between ticks and mites

Characters	**Ticks**	**Mites (parasitic)**
Size	Macroscopic	Microscopic
Eye	Usually, present	Usually, absent
Basis capituli	Well developed	Not well developed
Hair and bristles	Not prominent	Prominent
Respiration system	Trachea	Cuticle
Location	On skin	In skin
Life cycle	Do not spend entire life on host	Spend entire life on host

Suborder: Ixodida/Ixodoidea/Ixodides

1. This suborder is also known as **metastigmata** as the stigmata is of large size and present at the posterior part of the body.
2. Both males and females are blood suckers, however they can survive without food away from the hosts for a long period.

3. Suborder Ixodida is divided into two families: Argasidae (soft ticks) and Ixodidae (Hard ticks)

Characters	Argasidae (soft ticks)	Ixodidae (Hard ticks)
Dorsal shield/ Scutum	Dorsal shield is absent. A leathery and mammillated tegument is present on dorsal aspect in place of scutum.	A chitinous dorsal shield or scutum is present which extends over the whole dorsal surface of male and only a small portion behind the head in larvae, nymph and female.
Mouthparts	Mouthparts are ventral so not visible from the dorsal aspect.	Mouth parts are anterior so visible form both dorsal and ventral aspect.
Eyes	Eyes are either absent or there may be two pairs situated laterally on the supracoxal folds.	Eyes when present consist of one pair situated on the lateral margin of the scutum.
Spiracles	Spiracles present and located posterior to third pair of coxae.	Spiracles present and located posterior to fourth pair of coxae.
Festoon	Absent.	Usually present.
Sexual dimorphism	Indistinct.	Distinct.
Feeding habit	Nocturnal and intermittent feeder and take few minutes for complete feeding.	Feed day and night and take few days for complete feeding.
Mating	Mating off the host.	Mating on the host.
Life cycle	Eggs are laid in several batches after each blood meal. Usually, two nymphal stages are present.	Female lays all eggs in one batch only. Only one nymph stage is present.

Table: Characters of genera of ticks of veterinary importance

Size of Mouth Parts	Position of Mouth Parts	Other Characters	Genera Involved
Short	Ventral	Scutum absent Pulvilli absent Dorsal surface mammilated	*Argas* *Ornithodoros* *Otobius*
Long	Anterior	Pale rings on legs Eyes present and large	*Amblyomma* *Hyalomma*
Long	Anterior	Legs dark colour Eyes absent	*Ixodes*
Short	Anterior	Large eyes present Coxae I have paired spurs	*Dermacentor* *Rhipicephalus*
Short	Anterior	Eyes small or absent Coxae I have small paired or single spurs	*Boophilus* *Margaropus* *Haemaphysalis*

11

Soft Ticks (Argasidae)

Family: Argasidae

- The family includes fowl ticks and tampans.
- The integument is leather like, frequently mammillated and without dorsal shield.
- Capitulum and mouth parts are situated anteriorly and on ventral side, thus invisible from dorsal side.
- In general eyes are absent, if present these are two pairs and situated on lateral sides of supracoxal folds.
- Spiracles are one pair and situated posteriolaterally to the third coxae.
- Sexual dimorphism is not evident.
- The important genera are *Argas*, *Otobius* and *Ornithodoros*.

Genus: ***Argas***

Species: *Argas persicus*

Common name: Fowl Ticks

Host: Birds and sometimes man

Distribution: Worldwide

Morphological characters

- *Argas persicus* is perfectly oval with narrow anteriorly and broader posterior end.
- Length is 4 to 10 mm and width 2 to 6 mm.
- Lateral suture is present, mammillated integument texture.
- Engorge tick has slaty –blue colour while starved ones are yellowish – brown in colour.

- Sexes can be distinguished by the genital opening which is larger in the female than in male.

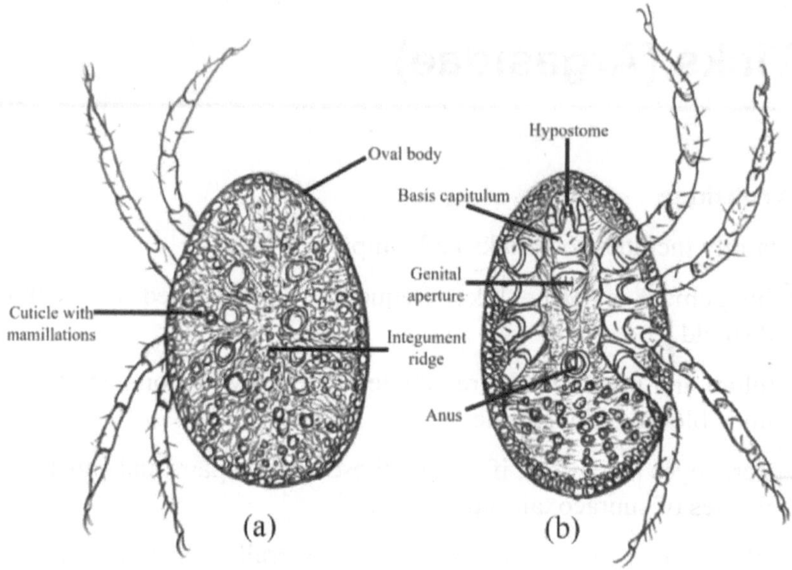

Figure 11.1. *Argas* (a) Dorsal (b) Ventral

Life cycle of *Argas persicus* (Fowl tick)

Female tick lays egg in cracks and crevices after blood meal. A female lays 20 to 100 eggs after each blood meal. Eggs are spherical and yellowish brown in colour. These eggs hatch after three weeks and larvae comes out. Larvae has got three pair of legs and mouth parts are located on anterior margin. Larvae are attached to body of host particularly on underside of the wing. They remain attached for five to ten days, during which they suck blood. After engorgement, they drop down and go to cracks and crevices, where they moult to nymphal stage in after seven days. Two nymph stage (Protonymph and deutonymph) are found in life cycle of *Argas persicus*. Each of which lasts for two weeks and feed only once particularly during night time. Then deutonymph moult to adult stage. All these moults occur off the host in cracks and crevices. Adult stages feed once in a month and after every blood meal they lay eggs in cracks and crevices. Adult ticks attach to body of bird during night time and feed for two hours.

Significance

1. **Anaemia:** All the stage of *Argas persicus* are blood suckers and heavily infested bird develops anaemia.
2. **Ticks worry:** Irritation caused by tick bite induces restlessness in birds which affects feeding and subsequently there is decrease in production.
3. **Ticks paralysis:** Saliva of tick is toxic giving rise to local inflammatory reaction and also induces paralysis in birds known as "tick paralysis".
4. **Vector of pathogen:** They transmit *Borrelia anserina,* etiological agent of "fowl spirochetosis" and *Aegypinella pullorum* in birds. *Argas* also transmit *Anapalsma marginale* in bovines.

Diagnosis: The ticks can be collected from cracks of woodworks and wall of poultry houses. The collected ticks are then identified by peculiar morphological characters.

Control

- The classical procedure includes removal of birds from poultry houses and placed in wooden crates for ten days for dropping of larvae from their body. Later the poultry is again put in cleaned and acaricide treated poultry house.
- Closure of cracks and crevices in poultry house.
- Spray or dusting of acaricides like organophosphates or synthetic pyrethroids in birds.
- Acaricidal spray in poultry house.

N.B: *Argas reflexus* is found on pigeons in India and other countries; it transmits *Borrelia anserina.*

Argas mainensis known as the Persainmaina bug and transmits relapsing fever in man.

Genus: *Otobius*

Species: *Otobius megnini*

Common name: Spinose ear tick

Host: Mainly dog but horse, bovines, sheep, goats, pigs, rabbit, wild animals and man.

Distribution: India, America and South Africa.

Morphological characters

- Approximately 6 mm in size.
- Integument texture have numerous spines like process, present on nymphal stage of tick which is bluish grey in color.
- Engorged larvae are almost spherical.
- **Nymph stage is widest at the middle. Adult has constriction at the middle, giving the body fiddle shaped.**

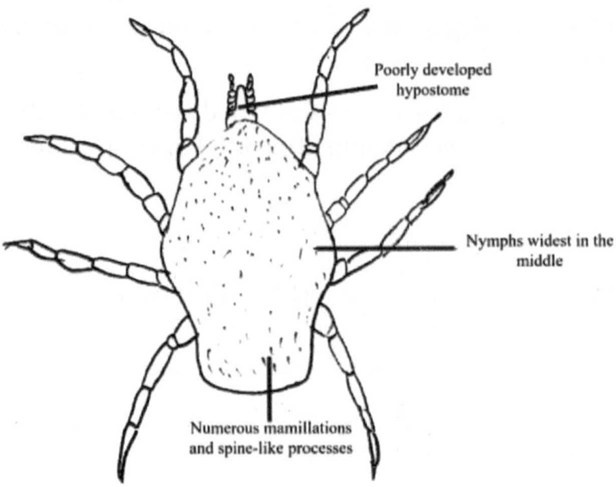

Figure 11.2. *Otobius* (Dorsal)

Life cycle: Adult ticks are not parasitic, but larval and nymphal stages are parasitic. Adult female lay 500-600 eggs in dark corners, crack and crevices of the animal house. These egg hatch in three to eight weeks and larvae come out and attached on body of host particularly of dog, horse, cattle and sheep and localized in ear particularly inner side of pinna where they survive for 2 to 3 months and feed on superficial lymph. Nymph stage is formed on body of host and survive for 7 to 10 months on ear. The fully engorged nymph drops down and seek for dry protective places like crevices and moult there to become adults (integument without spines).

Significance: Number of larvae and nymphs suck blood and produces marked irritation, this may result to inflammation in ears. Secondary bacterial infection may aggravate the condition. Infected dogs become dull, depressed, shake the head and scratch the infected ear. Waxy exudates is present in the ears. The condition is jointly termed as otitis. Fortunately, the tick doesn't transmit any disease except otitis in heavy infection.

Diagnosis: Presence of ticks in ear canal. In case of otitis a waxy exudate is removed to see the ticks in ear canal.

Treatment: Use of acaricides like synthetic pyrethroides into the ear to kill the stages of ticks.

Genus: *Ornithodoros*

Species: *Ornithodoros moubata*

Common name: Eyeless tampan of Africa

Host: Animals, poultry and man

Distribution: America and Africa. Not found in India

Morphological characters

- Adult are quite big (8 mm approx) as compared to *Argas* and *Otobius*.
- They are equally broad at anterior and posterior end.
- Other characters are similar but transverse groove present behind the 4th coxae.

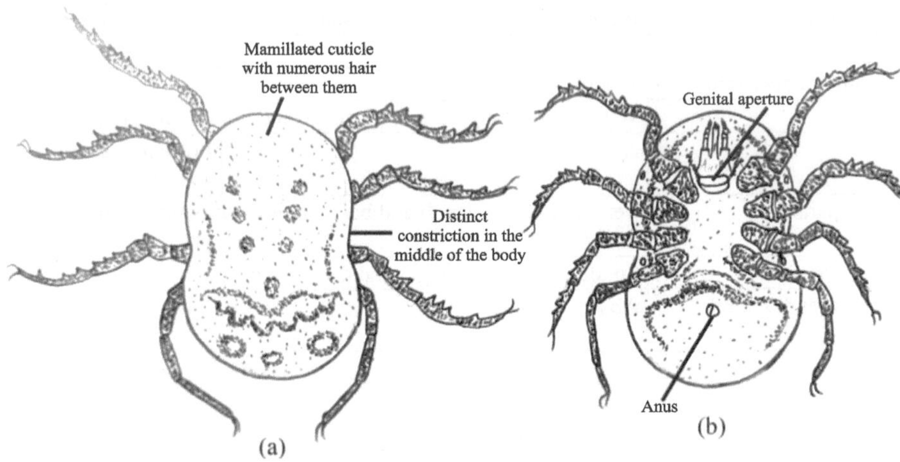

Figure 11.3. *Ornithodoros* (a) Dorsal (b) Ventral

Life cycle: A female lays batch of about 100 eggs in sand. Female broods eggs for eight days to hatch. The larvae remain quiescent until moult in nymphs. Several nymphal stages are present that attack the host for short period to feed only.

Significance: The nymphal and adult stage of ticks are parasitic but larval stage are not parasitic. It transmits spirochetosis (*Aegyptinella pullorum*) and *Borrelia anserina* in fowl, and anaplasmosis in animals. Tick is also reservoir host of African swine fever virus and vector of *Borrelia duttoni* (causes relapsing fever in human) and Q fever.

Control: Acaricide spray on walls of huts, animal buildings and houses. Application of acaricide like OP compounds and synthetic pyrethroids on animals and poultry as dust. Burning of house and rebuild it if animal house is made up of cheap replaceable materials like bamboo, palm mate etc.

N.B: *O. savignyi* is eye tampane found in India also. *O. turicata* is relapsing fever tick of USA. *O. lohorensis* is vector of *Theileria ovis* and *Anaplasma ovis* of goats and causes tick paralysis of sheep in Central Asia. *O. coriaceus* known as Pajaroello tick of cattle and deer in California and Pacific coast of Mexico. The tick bite is painful and causes epizootic bovine abortion in Central America.

Important morphological features of soft ticks

Features	*Argas*	*Otobius*	*Ornithodoros*
Size	6 mm		8 mm
Lateral suture	Present	Absent	Absent in nymph
Integument texture	Mammillated		Spined
Scutum or conscutum	Absent		
Legs	Without pale ring, slender in shape and pulvilli are absent		
Eyes	Absent		Present in some species
Mouth parts	Ventral, palp are small and basis capituli has straight lateral margins		
Spiracular plates	Small and between leg 3 and 4		
Festoons and Ventral plates	Absent in male		
Anal groove	Absent		
Coxae 1	Paired spurs absent		
Coxae 4	Normal in size		

12

Hard Ticks (Ixodidae)

Family: Ixodidae (Hard ticks)

General characters

- These ticks have hard chitinous shield called scutum on their dorsal surface, so they are called hard ticks. Scutum extends over the entire dorsal surface in male and only anterior one-third of dorsal surface in larvae, nymph and female.
- Mouth parts are anterior and visible from dorsal aspect.
- Eyes are one pair (if present) situated on the lateral margin of scutum.
- Spiracles are one pair and situated posterolaterally to the fourth coxae.
- Basis capituli or capitulum present at anterior, and have mouthparts and palps.
- The body of female may have one pair marginal grooves at lateral side of behind the scutum.
- Posterolateral and median grooves are present in both male and female on dorsal side.
- Posterior margin of ticks of some species is notched which is called **festoons** and is **generally eleven in number.**
- Certain species of ticks has coloured enamel like areas on the body, such ticks are called **ornate** ticks. Ticks which do not have enamel-like area are called **inornate** ticks.

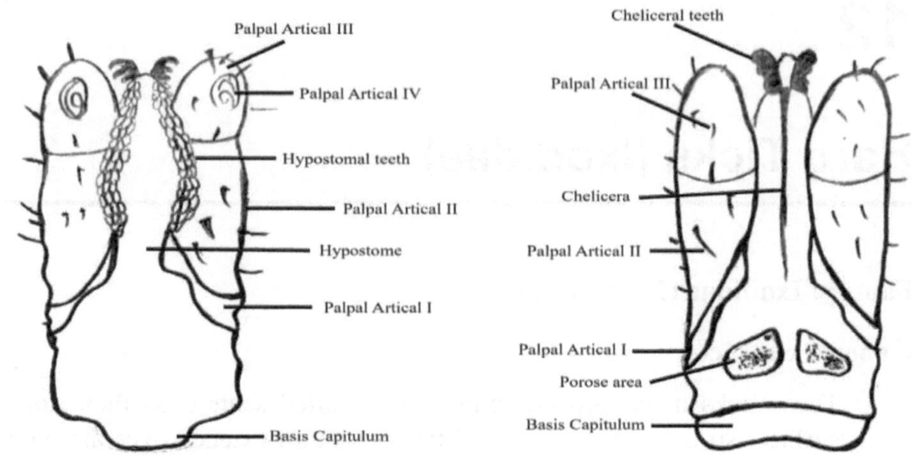

Figure 12.1. Mouth parts of ticks

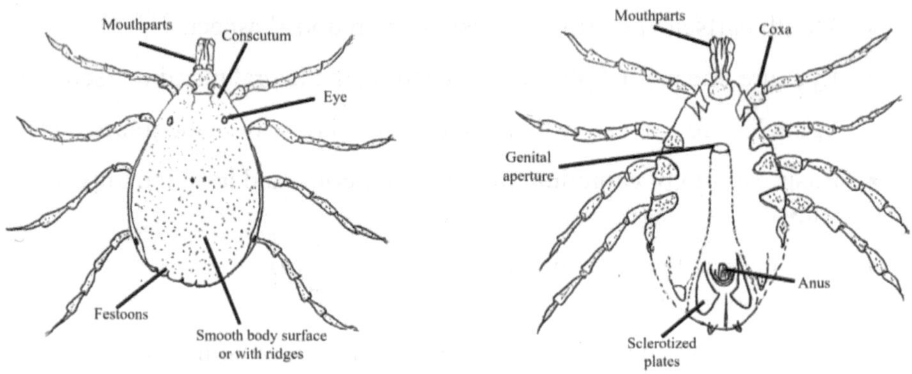

Figure 12.2. General morphology of male hard tick (a) Dorsal view (b) Ventral view

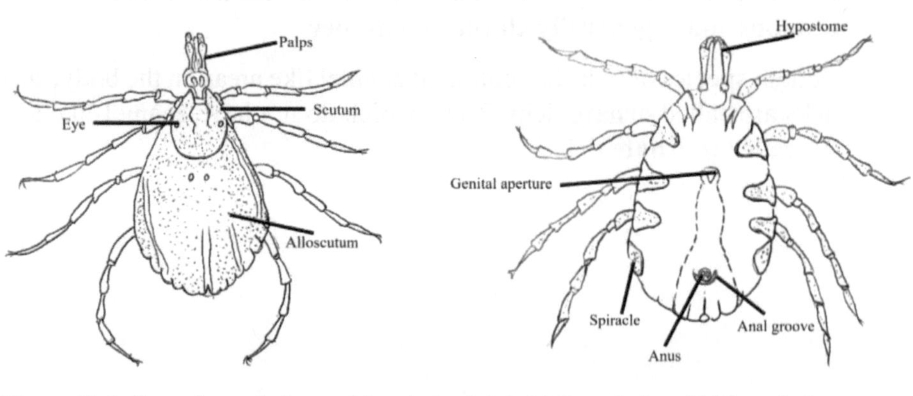

Figure 12.3. General morphology of female hard tick (a) Dorsal view (b) Ventral view

General Life Cycle

Ticks of family Ixodidae lay their eggs in sheltered spots or cracks and crevices in animal houses or ground. The eggs are laid in masses, and small, spherical in shape, yellowish brown to dark brown in colour. The female lays upto 18,000 eggs in a single batch and post which they die. The eggs hatch after certain period and larvae emerges. The newly hatched larvae are called **seed ticks** that climb up the grass or shrubs to wait for suitable host. The process of pre-oviposition period, hatching of eggs and development of different stages are greatly influenced by temperature and humidity. Larva moults into nymph and then imago/adult after engorgement on host. Copulation takes place on ground or on host. After copulation the female engorge on host and the drop down on ground and seek shelter space for egg laying. The male remains much longer time on their host. Depending upon number of hosts required by ticks for completion of its life cycle, ticks have been classified into three groups:

a) **One host tick:** All three instars engorge on the same animal and the moulting i.e. larve to nymph to imago takes place on the same host. e.g. *Boophilus annulatus*, *Boophilus decoloratus.*

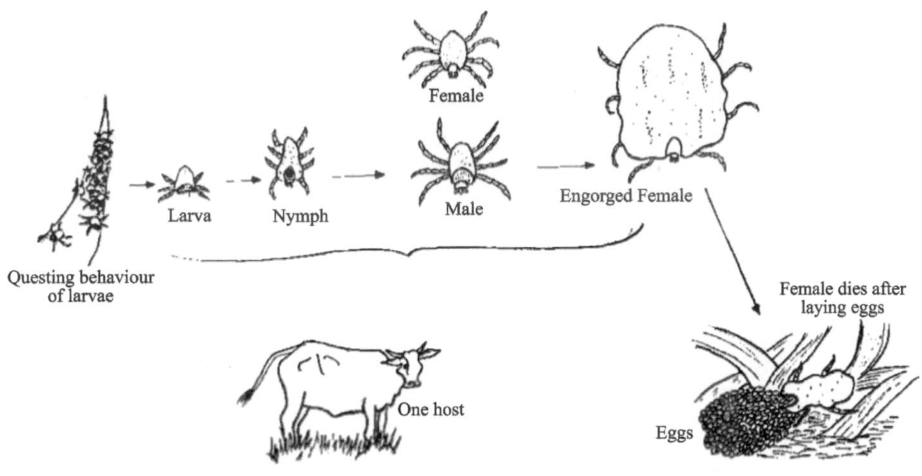

Figure 12.4 Life cycle of one host tick

b) **Two host tick:** There is requirement of two hosts to complete its lifecycle. The larva engorges and moults into nymph on the host. This nymph feed on same host and then drops down. The dropped, engorged nymph moult into imago on ground and seek new host for engorgement. e.g. *Rhipicephalus bursa*, *R. evertsi.*

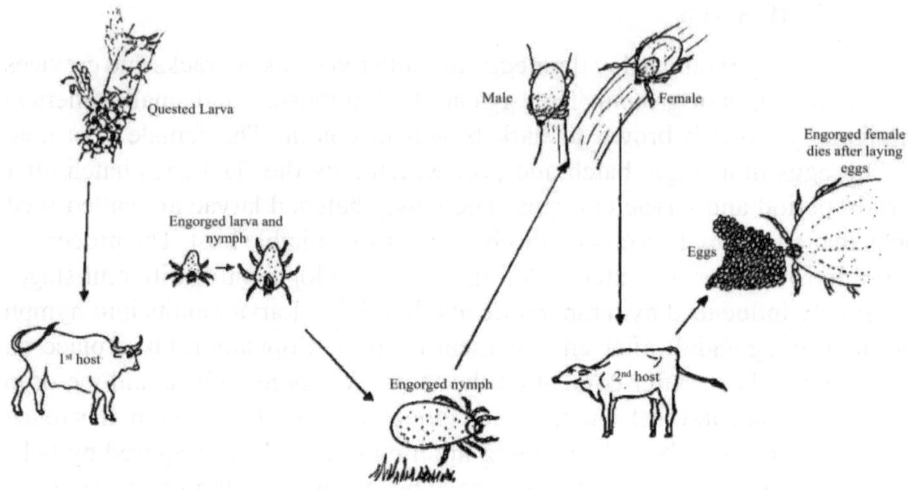

Figure 12.5. Life cycle of two host tick

c) **Three host tick:** The life cycle of three host tick completes in three hosts i.e. these ticks require a different host for every instar. Briefly, larva engorge on a host and drops down. This dropped larva moult in nymph on ground and attack on another host for feeding. After feeding on host again nymph drops down and moult into imago/adult. This imago/adult seek another host for feeding. That means a separate host is required for each developmental stage. e.g. *Rhipicephalus appendiculatus*, *Hyalomma anatolicum*, *Ixodes ricinus*.

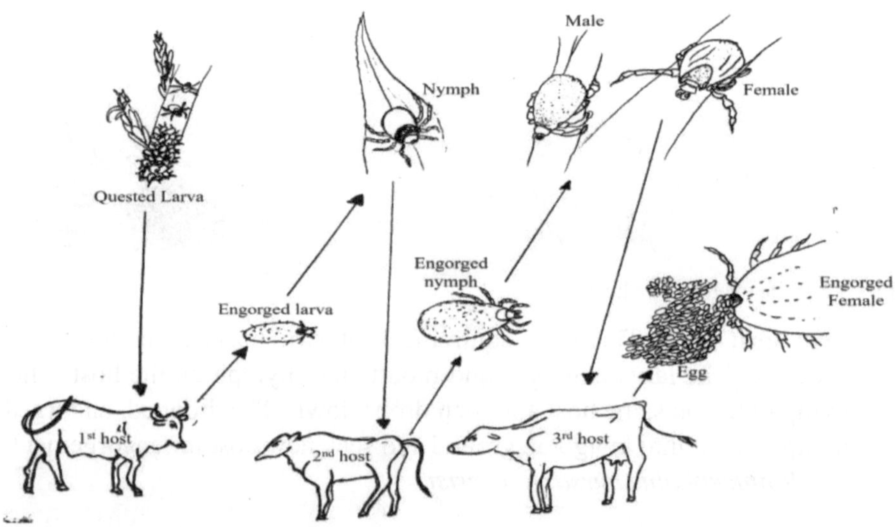

Figure 12.6. Life cycle of three host tick

Feeding Mechanism of Ticks

Tick buries its mouthparts into the host skin and remains attached on host during feeding. Due to host response during entering of tick mouth parts in host there is infiltration of neutrophils that causes destruction of collagen. This creates a cavity just below to mouth parts and is helpful to suck the blood directly.

Table: Key features of important Ixodid species

Genus	MP	Eye	Host	Basis capituli	Festoon	Ornate	Anal shield in Male
Boophilus	S	P	1	Hexagonal	A	A	P
Rhipicephalus	L	P	3	Hexagonal	P	A	P
Haylomma	L	P	2	Triangular	A/P	A	P
Haemaphysalis	S	A	3	Square	P	A	P
Ixodes	L	A	3	Square	A	A	P
Dermacentor	S	P	3	Square	P	P	A
Amblyomma	L	P	3	Square	P	P	A

MP = Mouth parts; S = small; L = large; P = present; A = absent; A/P = absent or present

Genus: *Ixodes*

Morphological characters

- Medium sized ticks of about 3-4 mm.
- Lateral suture absent, integument has striations.
- Palps are long.
- Basis capituli with straight lateral margins.
- Legs are slender and without pale rings. Pulvilli present.
- Eyes and festoons are absent.
- **Anal groove** surrounds the anus **anteriorly** and form a loop or circle.
- In male ventral surface bears a pregenital, median, anal, epidermal (paired) and adanal (paired) shields.
- Stigmatic plates are oval in male and circular in female.
- Coxae 4 are of normal size. Coxae 1 have unequal paired spurs.
- Three host tick.

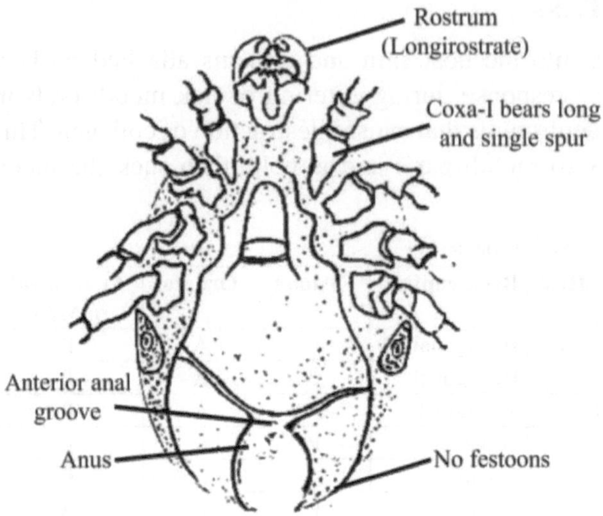

Figure 12.7. *Ixodes* spp. (Ventral view)

I. ricinus

- **Castor bean tick or sheep tick.** The dogs are major host but also reported from domestic and wild animals. The tick usually attached on less hairy regions like face, axillae and inguinal areas.
- Commonly distributed in Europe and Asia.
- The differential morphological characters include tarsi away to their ends and the posterolateral angle of Coxa I bears a spine which is long enough to overlap coxa II.
- *I. ricinus* transmits *B. divergens*, *B. bovis, Anaplasma marginale* in animals and looping ill virus, tick-borne fever, tick pyaemia in sheep.

I. rubicundus

- Paralysis tick of South Africa.
- Found on cattle, goats and sheep.
- *I. rubicundus* has morphological characters close to *I. pilosus*. The females have large white setae on the dorsal alloscutum which tend to give to the ticks a shining white appearance in both species. On *I. rubicundus* the setae are scattered over the dorsal alloscutum, on *I. pilosus* the setae are larger and occur in four columns. The scutum of females in *I. rubicundus* have a distinctly sinuous posterior margin

which often shows a distinct constriction. In *I. pilosus* the scutum have a slightly sinuous posterior margin. *I. rubicundus* has small auriculae on the ventral surface of the basis capituli, that are distinctly larger in *I. pilosus*. The anal groove in *I. rubicundus* extends to the posterior margin of the body as a long parallel pair of grooves compared to a short and converging pair in *I. pilosus*.

I. pilosus

- **Russet or sourveld or bush tick.**
- Found in S. Africa and affects cattle, sheep, goats, horses, dogs, cats and wild ruminants.

I. holocyclus

- Paralysis tick of Australia.
- Found on dogs, cat and other domestic animals.
- The species causes tick paralysis in dogs and transmits *Coxella burnetii.*

I. scapularis

- **Shoulder or black legged tick.**
- Found in North America and affects cattle, sheep, horse, dog and other animals.

I. pacificus

- **California black legged tick.**
- Found on cattle, sheep, goat and dogs.

Genus: *Rhipicephalus*

Morphological characters

- Size of unfed ticks is medium sizes of 3 to 5mm in size including mouthparts. Lateral suture is absent. Integument texture having striations.
- Palp articles are all small and basis capituli has distinct angular lateral margins to give a hexagonal shape of the entire basis capituli.
- Legs are slender, without pale rings except in *R. evertsi mimeticus.* Pulvilli are always present.

- Usually, inornate.
- Eyes present and flat to slightly convex (very convex or highly bulging in *R. evertsi*).
- Festoons are present but not clearly visible in engorged females.
- Spiracular plates are large and posterior to leg 4. Spiracle goblets are scattered over the spiracle plates. Spiracles are comma shaped short in female and long in male.
- Ventral plates (two) are present in males only.
- Anal groove is posterior to the anus.
- Coxae 4 are of normal size. Coxae I have large and paired spurs of equal size.
- Either two or three host tick.

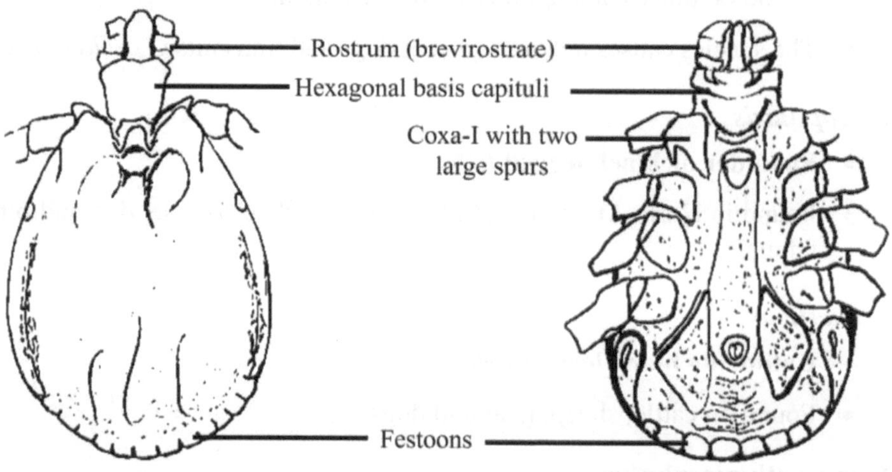

Figure 12.8. *Rhipicephalus* spp. (a) dorsal view (b) ventral view

R. appendiculatus

- Three host tick commonly known as **Brown ear tick** because of its colour and preference site for feeding on the ears of cattle.
- The tick affects cattle, horses, sheep, goats and dogs of Africa and other countries.
- The males have a prominent anterior spur on coxa I that is visible from the dorsal side. Have broader cervical fields with sharply raised margins,

fewer punctations, slightly convex eyes and the posterior grooves are not deeply sunken. The cervical fields in female are similar to the male, fewer punctations, slightly convex eyes and the genital pore is shallow V shape.

- The tick transmits *Theileria parva, T. taurotragi, T. mutans* and *B. bigemina, Anaplasma bovis* (*Ehrlichia bovis*) in cattle, *Hepatozoon canis* and exanthematic fever in dog, *Rickettsia conorii* in man, virus of Nairobi sheep disease and looping ill in sheep.

R. bursa

- Present in sheep, goats, cattle and horses of Europe, Africa and Asia.
- The male has a combination of an anterior spur on coxa I which is visible dorsally, a conscutum without apparent cervical fields, distinct lateral and posterior grooves, a densely punctate scutum and broad adanal plates. The scutum of the female is similar to the conscutum of the male in being densely punctate and without apparent cervical fields. Both sexes have a highly characteristic concentration of setae around the spiracles.
- Tick transmits *Babesia bigemina* and *Babesia bovis* to cattle, *Babesia caballi* and *Theileria equi* (= *Babesia equi*) in horses, and *Babesia ovis* to sheep. It also transmits *Anaplasma marginale, Rickettsia ovina, Coxiella burnetii* and virus of Nairobi sheep disease.

Rhipicephalus evertsi evertsi

- It is two host tick commonly known as the **red-legged tick**.
- It is widely distributed and common on domestic and wild animals throughout much of Africa and also reported from USA.
- This is the largest *Rhipicephalus* species having two sub-species ***Rhipicephalus evertsi evertsi*** and ***R. evertsi mimeticus***. They have very convex beady eyes and the scutum is covered with many punctations. *R. evertsi evertsi* have uniform orange-coloured legs while *R. evertsi. mimeticus* has yellow rings on its legs. The rings, the large size and the feeding site of the adult ticks may lead to confusion between *R. evertsi. mimeticus* and *Hyalomma* ticks, but the mouthparts of the *R. evertsi. mimeticus* are short compared to the long mouthparts in *Hyalomma* ticks.

Rhipicephalus sanguineus

- It is three host tick commonly known as the **kennel tick or the pan-tropical dog tick or Brown dog tick**.
- The tick is cosmopolitan in distribution on dogs.
- The tick is dull yellow colour to mid brown colour. The genital aperture is usually a broad U-shaped. Spiracle plates are narrow with tails that is less than the width of the adjacent festoon in both sexes. Depression of the cervical fields are absent in male.
- The tick transmits *Ehrlichia canis, Babesia canis, Babesia gibsoni* and *Hepatozoon canis* in dogs and *Rickettsia conorii* in man.

Sub-Genus: *Boophilus*

The *Boophilus* sub-genus comes within the genus *Rhipicephalus* are so well known in their original classification, as members of the full genus *Boophilus* that the former names are likely to remain in use for some time without confusion. The characterisitcs that have been used for this sub-genus are separate from the rest of the genus *Rhipicephalus*.

Morphological characters

- Size of unfed ticks is about 2 to 3mm, lateral suture is absent. Integument texture has striations.
- Palps are small with prominent transverse ridges. Basis capituli has angular lateral margins.
- Legs are slender and without pale rings. Pulvilli are always present.
- Scutum present and without enamel.
- Eyes are present but indistinct.
- Festoons absent.
- Spiracular plates are large and posterior to leg 4. Spiracle goblets are scattered over the spiracle plates.
- Ventral plates are present in males only.
- Anal groove is indistinct, if visible it is posterior to the anus.
- Coxae IV are of normal size. Small paired spurs present on Coxae I (bifid).

- Genital aperture of females is a small U or V shaped.
- One host tick.

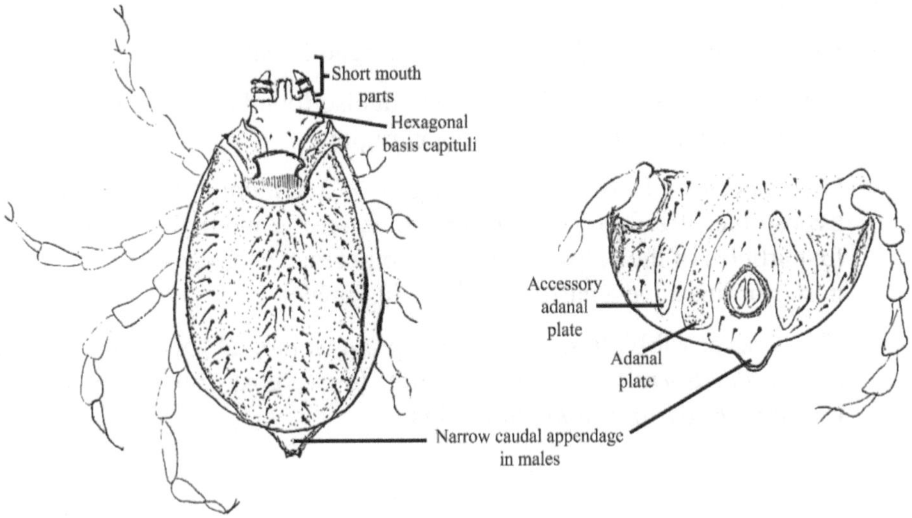

Figure 12.9. *Boophilus* sp.

B. microplus

- **Tropical cattle tick**.
- Affects cattle but also sheep, goats and deers.
- *Rhipicephalus* (*B.*) *microplus* has 4 + 4 columns of teeth on its hypostome. Has no protuberance bearing setae on the inner margin of palp. Caudal appendage present.
- The tick is responsible for transmission of *Babesia bigemina*, *Borrelia theileri* and *Anaplasma*.

B. annulatus

- North American tick.
- Affects domestic and wild ungulates of America and Africa.
- The hypostomal teeth are in 4 + 4 columns. The internal margin of the first palp article is long and slightly concave. The spurs and cleft between the spurs on the first coxa of females are less distinct. The second coxa of females is without a spur. A caudal appendage in male is absent. The shape of porose area at basis capituli is a broad oval.

- The tick is responsible for transmission of *Babesia bigemina, Borrelia theileri* and *Anaplasma.*

B. decoloratus

- **Blue tick** because of the colour of engorged females.
- Cattle and equines are primary host but also found in sheep, goats, wild ungulate and also in dog of Ethopian region.
- Only species of *Boophilus* having 3 + 3 columns of teeth on the hypostome. Presence of a protuberance on the internal margin of the first articles of the palps that bears two pectinate setae. Genital aperture posterior lips have a narrow U shape in female.
- The tick possibly transmits *Babesia bigemina, B. ovis, Anaplasma marginale, Borrelia theileri* in cattle, horse, goat and sheep. It also transmits *Babesia trautmanii* in pigs.

B. geigyi

- Tick affects cattle sheep and wild ungulates and confined in only West Africa.
- Morphologically similar to *B. decoloratus* except 4 + 4 columns of teeth present on the hypostome and genital aperture posterior lips have a narrow V-shape in female.
- The transmission of pathogen by this tick is not known.

Genus: *Margaropus*

Morphological characters

The characters of this genus are similar to sub-genus *Boophilus* except-

- Size about 3mm including mouthparts.
- Legs are bulbous (very bulbous in males).
- The adanal plates are distinctly long and sharp.
- The medial ventral plate is prolonged into two spines, projecting either side of anus.
- The genital aperture of females is wide and oval in shape.
- Coxa I have small posterior spine.
- One host tick.

Margaropus winthemi

- Commonly known as **Argentine tick or winter horse tick, or South African beady-legged tick**.
- Found on horses and cattle, and distributed in America and Africa.
- Legs are thick as compare to *R. (B.) decoloratus* and have dark bands at joints of legs. *Margaropus winthemi* infest horse in winter.
- Do not transmit any pathogens.

Margaropus reidi

- It is **Sudanese beady-legged tick** found on Giraffe in West Sudan.
- Other characters are similar to *M. winthemi*.

Genus: *Hyalomma*

Morphological characters

- Large sized tick of about 5 to 6 mm including mouthparts. Lateral suture is absent. Striations present on integument.
- Palp articles 2 are longer than articles 1 and 3.
- Basis capituli has medium angular lateral margins.
- Legs are slender and usually have pale rings. Pulvilli are always present.
- Scutum or conscutum have brown coloured. Enamel is usually absent (inornate) from the scutum.
- ***H. lusitanicum* is an ornate tick.**
- Eyes are always present and very convex.
- Festoons are present.
- Spiracular plates are large and posterior to fourth legs. Spiracle goblets are scattered over the spiracle plates. Spiracles are comma shaped in males and triangular in male.
- Three ventral plates are present in only males.
- Anal groove is posterior to the anus.
- Coxae IV are of normal size. Coxae I have large and equal paired spurs.

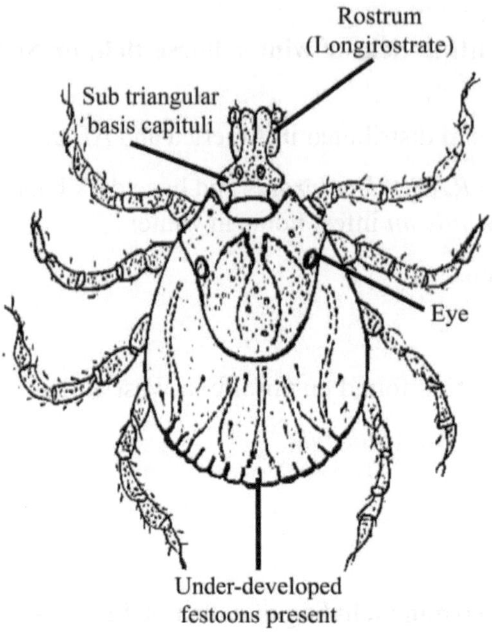

Figure 12.10. *Hyalomma* spp. (dorsal view)

Hyalomma anatolicum anatolicum

- Two-host tick on hares and three-host tick on cattle.
- Adults feed on cattle, sheep, goats, camels, horses and donkeys in North Africa to India.
- The females have shallower cervical fields with parallel sides.
- The males have a less distinctly depressed area at the posterior of the scutum and the paracentral festoons are not joined anteriorly to form an arch.
- The tick species transmits *Theileria annulata, Theileria lestoquardi, Theileria equi, Babesia caballi, Trypanosoma theileri* causing benign bovine and Crimean-Congo haemorrhagic fever virus.

Hyalomma anatolicum excavatum

- Two-host or three-host tick depending on availability of hosts.
- It is a robust and approximately 25% larger than *H. anatolicum anatolicum*, dark in colour with the ringed legs. In females the shape of cervical fields has steep sides and curved margins. The males have a

distinctive depressed area in the posterior scutum, with steep sides. They have a distinctive formation of the festoons such that the paracentral festoons are joined anteriorly to form an arch, also the central festoon is pale.

- The tick act as a vector of *Theileria.*

Other species are *H. plumbeum plumbeum* in Southern Europe, *H. detrittum scupense*, *H. detritum mauretanicum* in North Africa.

Genus: *Haemaphysalis*

Morphological characters

- Small sized ticks of about 3mm including mouthparts. Lateral suture is absent and striations present on integument.
- Palps usually short and conical (in some species), Palp articles 2 are usually broad and having conspicuous projection.
- Basis capituli has straight lateral margins.
- Legs are slender and without pale rings. The trochanter of first pair of legs has a dorsal process. Pulvilli are always present.
- Inornate tick.
- Eyes are always absent.
- Festoons are present.
- Spiracular plates are large and posterior to legs 4. Spiracle goblets are scattered over the spiracle plates. Spiracles in female is oval or comma shaped while oval in male.
- Ventral plates are absent from males.
- Anal groove is posterior to the anus.
- Coxa IV are of normal size. Coxae I have unequal paired spurs (only a single internal spur is present).

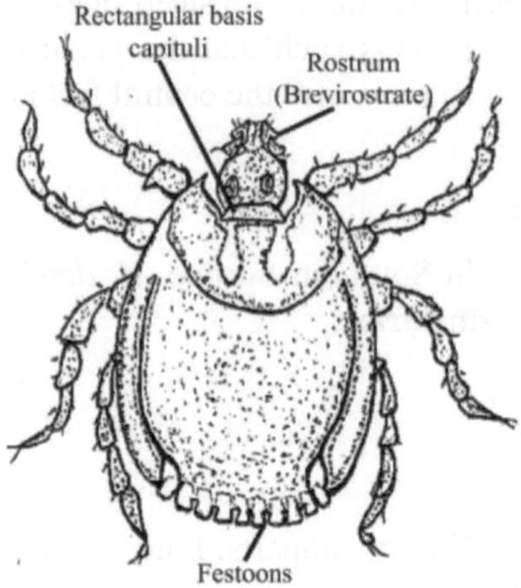

Figure 12.11. *Haemaphysalis* spp. (dorsal view)

Haemaphysalis leachi

- Three host tick commonly known as the **yellow dog tick**.
- Affects wild and domestic carnivores of Africa, Australia and Asia.
- Tick has conspicuous lateral extensions to palp articles 2, forming mouthparts with a distinctive conical shape.
- The coxa IV of males have only medium length spurs.
- It transmits *Babesia canis* in dog, *Rickettsia conorii* and *Coxiella brunetii* to humans.

Haemaphysalis punctata

- Three host tick known as **red sheep tick**.
- Affects sheep, goat, deer, cattle in Europe, Japan and North Africa.
- The palp articles 2 with only a small lateral extension the mouthparts do not form the distinctly conical shape.
- The females have 11 festoons from this three are enclosed by the lateral groove on each side (visible when the specimen is unfed). The females also have medium size spurs on coxae I to III.
- The tick transmits *Babesia motasi* and possibly other species of *Babesia*. It also transmits *Theileria ovis* and *Theileria buffeli* and anaplasmosis.

H. leporis-palustri

- Three host tick commonly known as **rabbit tick**.
- Found chiefly in rabbit of USA.
- It transmits *Coxiella brunetii*, Rocky Mountain spotted fever and Tularemia fever in man.

***H. chordelis*:** Commonly known as bird tick. Chiefly found in birds in North and South America.

H. humerosa: Found in bandicoots in Australia

H. longicornis

- Known as **Bush tick or New Zealand tick**.
- Occurs in man cattle, sheep, goat and birds in Japan, China, Australia and New Zealand.
- The tick transmits *Theileria* and *Coxiella brunetii.*

Genus: *Dermacentor*

Morphological characters

- Medium sized ticks of about 4 to 5 mm (*D. nitens* is about 3mm).
- Lateral suture is absent. Striations on integument.
- Palps are short. Palp articles 2 are broad (small in *D. nitens*).
- Basis capituli is rectangular has straight lateral margins.
- Legs are slender without pale rings. Pulvilli are always present.
- Enamel (ornamentation) usually present on scutum and conscutum in a white pattern (absent in *D. nitens*).
- Eyes are present and usually flat to slightly convex (indistinct in *D. nitens*).
- Festoons are present.
- Spiracular plates are large and posterior to legs 4. Spiracle goblets are scattered over the spiracle plates (form a ring in *D. nitens*).
- Ventral plates are absent from males.
- Anal groove is posterior to the anus (indistinct in *D. nitens*).

- Coxae IV are very large. Coxae I is bifid and have large and equal paired spurs.

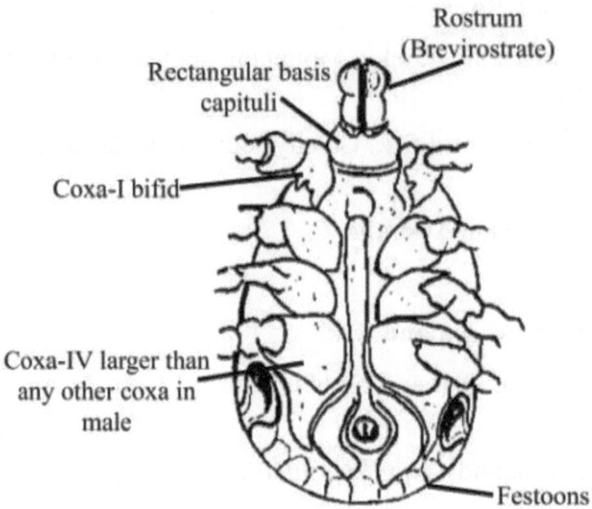

Figure 12.12. *Dermacentor* spp. (ventral view)

Dermacentor marginatus

- Three host tick commonly known as the **ornate sheep tick**.
- Affects cattle, sheep, goats and dogs in Africa, Iran, Afganistan.
- Characteristically white enamel present on the scutum or conscutum with other genera characters.
- It transmits *Babesia canis* to dogs and *Rickettsia conorii* to humans.

D. reticulates

- Three host tick distributed in USSR, Central Europe, France and England in many domestic and wild animals.
- It transmits *B. equi* and *B. canis*.

D. andersoni

- Three host tick known as **Rocky Mountain wood tick**
- Affects variety of mammals in USA and known as primary vector of *Rickettsia rickettsii*.

- It also transmits *Anaplasma, Babesia canis, Leptospira pomona* and *Coxiella brunetii.*

D. nitens

- One host tick known as the **tropical horse tick**.
- Affects equines and sheep, cattle and goat of Mexico, Florida, South America and USA.
- It transmits equine piroplasmosis also causes suppuration of ears.

D. albipictus

- **Winter or moose tick** of moose also found in sheep, goat and wild animals, distributed in North USA.
- It transmits anaplasmosis and Rocky Mountain spotted fever.

D. occidentalis

- Three host tick known as **Pacific coast tick**.
- Affects sheep, donkey, horse, rabbit and man in Pacific coast of California.
- Transmits *Anaplasma*, Colorado tick fever, Q fever and tularaemia.

D. nigrolineatus

- One host tick known as **brown winter tick**.
- Affects wild tailed deer, horses and cattle in USA.

Genus: *Amblyomma*

Morphological characters

- Size of tick is about 6 to 7 mm.
- Lateral suture is absent. Striations on integument.
- Hypostome and palpi are long. Palp articles 2 are longer than articles 1 and 3.
- Basis capituli has straight lateral margins.
- Legs are slender, usually have pale rings. Pulvilli are always present.
- Enamel (ornamentation) is present on the scutum.

- Eyes are always present and may be flat or convex.
- Festoons are present.
- Spiracular plates are large and posterior to legs. Spiracle goblets are scattered over the spiracle plates.
- Ventral plates in males are indistinct and in the form of small flat chitinous plaques posterior to the anus. The ventral surface of the festoons has plates known as scutes.
- Anal groove is posterior to the anus.
- Coxae IV are of normal size. Coxae I have unequal paired spurs.

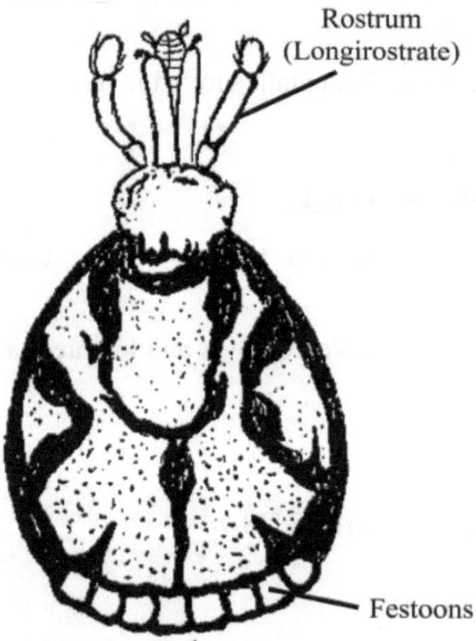

Figure 12.13. *Amblyomma* spp. (dorsal view)

Amblyomma hebraeum

- Three-host tick, known as the **South African bont tick**.
- Affects cattle, sheep, goats, large wild ruminant and birds of USA and Africa.
- Tick has flat eyes close to the margin of scutum.
- The female has complex pattern of enamel but without connections between the central and lateral spots. The male has distinctive enamel ornamentation on 9 of 11 festoons.

- The species transmits *E. ruminantium, Theileria mutans, Rickettsia conorii* and *Rickettsia africae.*

Amblyomma variegatum

- A three-host tick, known as the **tropical bont tick or variegated tick**, affects cattle, sheep, goats and other herbivores of Africa.
- Tick has distinctly convex eyes which are separated from the margin of the scutum, Males have an enamel pattern usually without lateral spots and there is no enamel on the festoons.
- The enamel of both sexes is pink to orange in colour.
- The tick responsible for the transmission of *Ehrlichia ruminantium* (= *Cowdria ruminantium*), *Ehrlichia bovis, Theileria mutans, Theileria velifera* and *Coxiella brunetii.*

Amblyomma americanum

- A three-host tick, known as **lone star tick**.
- Affects variety of animals of USA.
- A single large white spot present on the scutum of female.
- The tick transmits Q fever, Rocky Mountain spotted fever and tularemia fever.

Amblyomma cajennense

- A three-host tick, known as **cayenne tick**.
- Affects horses and other animals of South and Central America.
- The species transmits *Leptospira pomona*, fever and death to cattle.

Amblyomma maculatum

- A three-host tick, known as **Gulf Coast tick**.
- Affects cattle, sheep, goat, horse and man of Gulf of Mexico.
- Bite of tick is painful also causes tick paralysis.

Genus: *Aponomma*

Morphological characters

- Almost similar to *Amblyomma*
- Eyes are vestigial or absent.
- The host are reptiles.

Genus: *Rhipicentor*

Morphological characters

- Closely resemble to Genus *Dermacentor*
- Enamel absent, Inornate tick.
- Basis caputuli hexagonal dorsally with prominent lateral angle.
- Coxa IV in male bears two spurs.
- Ticks found in Africa.
- Species ***Rhipicentor bicorinis*** (found in different animals) and ***R. nuttalli*** (hedgehogs, dogs, and cattle).

Table: Important distinguishing characters of important hard ticks

Genus	Species of ticks	Type of tick	Morphological characters	Significance/Vector of disease
Ixodes			Inornate, Eyes and festoon absent, Longirostrate (mouthparts longer), Stigmatic plates oval in male, circular in female.	
	Ixodes ricinus (Castor bean tick)	Three host tick	The posterolateral angle of Coxa I bears a spine which is long enough to overlap coxa II.	1. *Babesia* 2. *Anaplasma*
	Ixodes holocyclus	Three host tick	-	Tick paralysis
	Ixodes scapularis (Shoulder tick or black legged tick)	Three host tick	-	-
Hyalomma (Bont legged tick)			Inornate, Eyes present, Festoon usually present, basis capituli triangular, longirostrate, spiracles comma shape in male and triangular in female. Legs have rings of white pigment at the far end of segment.	
	Hyalomma anatolicum anatolicum	Three host tick	Festoon present	1.*Theileria annulata* 2. *Theileria equi* 3.Congo hemorrhagic fever
Rhipicephalus			Inornate, Eyes present, festoon usually present, brevirostrate (mouthparts smaller), basis capituli hexagonal.	
	Rhipicephalus (Boophilus) microplus (Tropical cattle tick)	One host tick	Festoon absent, palps with prominent transverse ridges. Coxa I bifid. Parasitic period on host is 17-52 days.	1. *Babesia* 2. *Anaplasma*
	Rhipicephalus appendiculatus (Brown ear tick)	Three host tick	Festoon present	1. *Theileria parva* 2. *Hepatozoon canis* 3. *Babesia* 4. Ticks toxicosis

Genus	Species of ticks	Type of tick	Morphological characters	Significance/Vector of disease
	Rhipicephalus sanguineus (Brown dog tick)	Three host tick	Festoon present	1. *Babesia caballi* 2. *Babesia equi* 3. *Babesia canis* 4. *Babesia vogeli* 5. *Babesia gibsoni* 6. *Anaplasma marginale* 7. *Hepatozoon canis* 8. *Ehrlichia canis*
	Rhipicephalus evertsi (Red legged tick)	Two host tick	Festoon present	1. *Theileria parva* 2. *Theileria mutans* 3. *Babesia bigemina*
	Rhipicephalus bursa	Two host tick	Festoon present	1. *Babesia ovis* 2. *Babesia caballi* 3. *Babesia equi*
Haemaphysalis			Inornate, eyes absent, festoon present, palps short and conical, brevirostrate, basis capituli rectangular, ventral surface without chitinous plates.	
	Haemaphysalis leachi (Yellow dog tick)	Three host tick	-	*Babesia canis*
	Haemaphysalis spinigera	Three host tick	-	KFD (Kyasanur forest disease)
Dermacentor			Usually ornate, basis capituli rectangular, eyes and festoon present, brevirostrate, hypostome and palps short , Coxa I bifid, and coxa IV of male is much longer than coxa I to III. No plate on ventral surface of male.	

Genus	Species of ticks	Type of tick	Morphological characters	Significance/Vector of disease
	Dermacentor andersoni	Three host tick	-	1. *Babesia canis* 2.*Anaplasma marginale* 3.*Rickettsi rickettssii* (rocky mountain spotted fever) 4.Western equine encephalomyelitis 5.*Coxiella burnetii* 6. Tick paralysis
	Dermacentor nitens (Tropical horse tick)	One host tick	-	1.Equine babesiosis
Amblyomma			Usually ornate, eyes and festoon present, longirostrate, male without ventral plates but small chitinous plaques may be present. The species are usually large and broad.	
	Amblyomma hebraeum (Bont tick	Three host tick	-	*Rickettsia ruminantium*
	Amblyomma variegatum (Tropical bont tick or variegated tick)	Three host tick	-	Heart water disease
	Amblyomma americanum (Lone star tick)	Three host tick	-	-
Aponomma (reptile ticks)		One host tick	Eyes present, ornate, festoon present, longirostrate.	-
Nosomma		Three host tick	Eyes present, brevirostrate.	

Pathogenic significance of ticks

1. **Injury to skin through bites**: Biting by tick cause wounds on the skin. The wounds may predispose the secondary bacterial infection in hot and humid climate that may lead to formation of pustules and suppuration. The wounds are also made susceptible to host to attract and attack of blow flies and screw worm flies. Similarly, if wounds are created on soft or delicate skin, severe inflammatory reactions occur particularly on udder, that makes milking very difficult. Infestation of large number of ticks cause injury to the skin which in turn reduce the quality and deprecation of the hide.

2. **Blood sucking habits leading to anemia**: A single female tick takes around 0.5-2ml of blood during it's stay on the body of host, likewise hundreds of ticks are present on body of host and may lead to severe blood loss causing anaemia.

3. **Death of animals:** Thousands of ticks on body of animals causes severe blood loss and may lead to death to animals.

4. **Tick worry:** The infestation with few hundred ticks on animals is usual in nature, it produces comparatively less harmful effect in a condition "tick worry". This includes combination of different entities like irritation, secondary attack by flies and bacteria and blood loss results in improper feed intake by animals leading to reduced milk production and decrease body growth.

5. **Tick paralysis:** This is characterized by **acute ascending flaccid motor paralysis** caused by the release toxins of adults and nymphal stages during feeding. Ticks primarily responsible ticks for paralysis are: *Argas persicus, Ornithodoros lahorensis, Dermacentor andersoni* and *Ixodes holocyyclus*. Degree of paralysis is directly proportional to the number of ticks, duration of time of attachment of ticks and location of ticks on body of animal. Likewise, animal is more susceptible to paralysis if ticks are attached close to head and vertebral column. Condition may become fatal when respiratory muscles are involved. However, toxin causing paralysis is reversible and has very short shelf life. If the ticks are removed in time, toxin metabolizes and is excreted out from the body thereby recovering animal from paralysis. Recovered animals become immune to the toxins of the ticks.

6. **Tick toxicosis:** It is a distinctive form of tick paralysis and caused by toxin released by specific species of ticks. Sweating sickness in

Africa and India by toxin of *Hyalomma* in ruminants and pigs during summer is the best example among different tick toxicosis. The toxin is antigenically and chemically different from toxin which causes paralysis and causes profuse moist eczema and hyperaemia of mucous membrane that may lead to death of young ones.

Another type of toxin is leucocytotropic toxin produced by *Rhipicephalus appendiculatus*, which has been reported in Africa.

7. **Disease transmission:** Different species of ticks are responsible for transmission of disease producing organisms like virus, bacteria, protozoa and rickettsia has already been mentioned.

Control of Ticks

1. Application of Acaricides: The knowledge of biology of different ticks is essential for effective control. This include one/two/three host tick, duration of tick season during which the ticks are present on the body of host or in cracks and crevices. **One host tick is easier to control than three host ticks**. Different methods of application are dusting, sprays, pour-on and dips.

a. Organaphosphate compounds like Malathion, Sumithion @ 0.05%
b. Pyrethroides: Cypermethrin/Deltamethrin @ 2- 3 ml. of this solution in one liter of water effective.
c. Formamidines: Amitraz® @ 3 ml in 1 liter of water.
d. lvermectin @ 300 - 400 μg per kg body weight S/C at weekly interval. But drug of choice is Amitraz® @ 3 ml in 1 liter of water. If secondary bacterial invasion, give antibiotics and supportive treatment with corticosteroides and antihistaminic agents to avoid itiching.
e. Phytoacaricides: Neem oil, Karanj oil.

Before application of the acaricides, animal body must be cleaned of dust and dirt. Also, animal should be given water and be prevented from licking the skin after spraying.

2. Pasture management

a. **Rotational grazing or pasture spelling**: Animals are not allowed to graze in the infected pasture for a long period. As a result, ticks and their stages die of starvation.
b. **Burning of pasture**: Burning may kill ticks and their stages which are present on pastures or in soil.

c. **Ploughing of land**: Ploughing of land will expose the ticks to the harsh sunlight or they will be buried deep in the soil and get killed.

3. Biological Control

a. **Plants:** Plants like *Melinis, Cynodon* are having repellant activity. Tropical legume of genus *Stylosanthes* produce sticky substance which immobilize and kill the ticks.

b. **Insects:** Hymenopterous flies are natural enemies of ticks, for instance, ixodiphagous (e.g. *Hunterellus*), they parasitize especially the nymph in which they lay eggs and which are literally eaten out by the larvae of parasite. Fire ant predates on ticks like *Amblyomma* spp.

c. **Birds:** Some birds (e.g. *Bubulcus ibis*) destroy the ticks.

d. **Bacteria: e.g.** *Bacillus thurungiensis*, when ingested by ticks, act as stomach poison.

e. **Fungi:** Fungus *Aspergillus flavus*, *Beuveria* spp. multiply and grow on tick cuticle and cause damage.

4. Immunological control: Recombinant vaccine containing midgut protein Bm86 against *Rhipicephalus* (*Boophilus*) *microplus* and available commercially as Tickgard® (Australia) and Gavac® (Cuba) has been expressed in *Escherichia coli* and *Pichia pastoris* respectively. Another vaccine, Tick gard Plus® containing mid gut antigen Bm86 and salivary gland antigen Bm91 has been developed with higher efficacy.

However, these vaccines are not effective in most of other parts of world including India due to strain variation.

5. Genetic control: Various breeds are being screened and evaluated for development of tick resistant breed of animals. *Bos indicus* is relatively resistant than *Bos taurus* to ticks infestation.

6. Sterile Male technique: Cross between two species of ticks like *Rhipicephalus* (*Boophilus*) *microplus* and *Rhipicephalus* (*Boophilus*) *annulatus* will produce sterile male offsprings and hybrid females which will produce hybrid females in three back-cross generations.

13

Mites

Mites

Subclass: Acari

Order: Parasitiformes

Suborder: Gamasida/Mesostigmata

Characters

1. Mites of this group have the stigmata or spiracles in the middle of the body, hence suborder Gamasida is also called suborder mesostigmata. Mites of this group are referred as gamasid mite.
2. Size of these mites are large about 0.6-2.5 mm in length and hence visible via naked eye.
3. They parasitisize birds and mammals.

Important genera and species

1. Genus: *Dermanyssus*

Species: *Dermanyssus gallinae*

Host: Birds rarely feed on man

Common name: **Red mite of poultry**

Distribution: Cosmopolitan

Morphological Characters

1. Mites look like spider.
2. Chelicerae are long and whiplike.

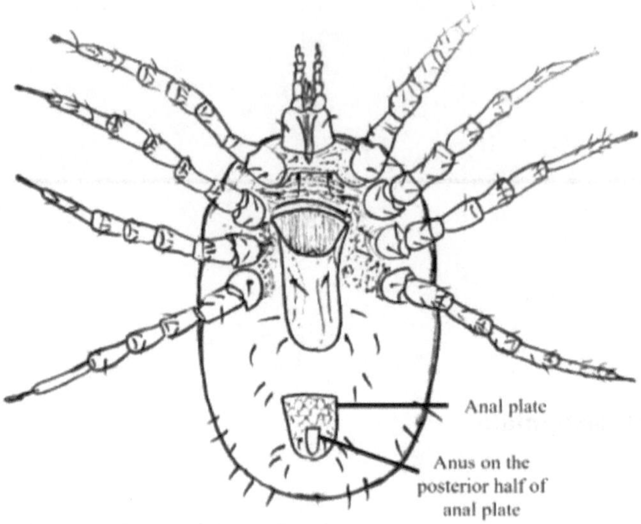

Figure 13.1. *Dermanyssus gallinae*

Significance

1. They suck blood.
2. They transmit *Borrelia anserina,* causative agent of spirochetosis of fowl.
3. They cause skin lesions in human being.

2. Genus: *Ornithonyssus*

- **Species:** *Ornithonyssus sylviarum*

Host: Birds

Common name: Northern mite of poultry

- **Species:** *Ornithonyssus bacoti*

Host: Rats and man

Common name: Tropical rat mite

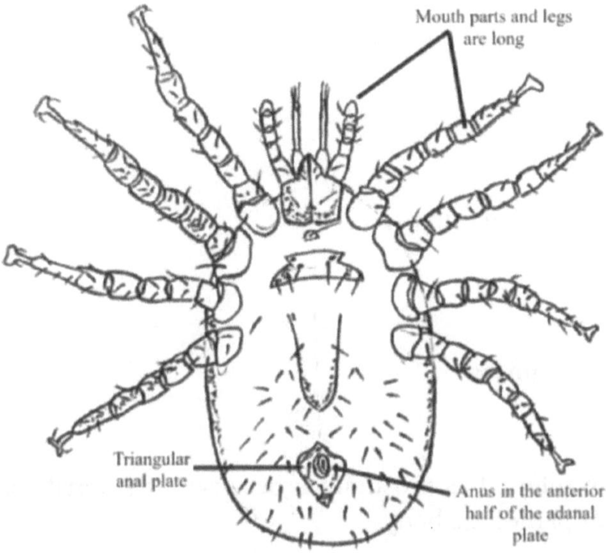

Figure 13.2. *Ornithonyssus*

3. Genus: *Pneumonyssus*

Species: *Pneumonyssus caninum*

Host: Dog

Significance: Lives in the nasal passages and nasal sinuses of the dog and cause rhinitis and sinusitis.

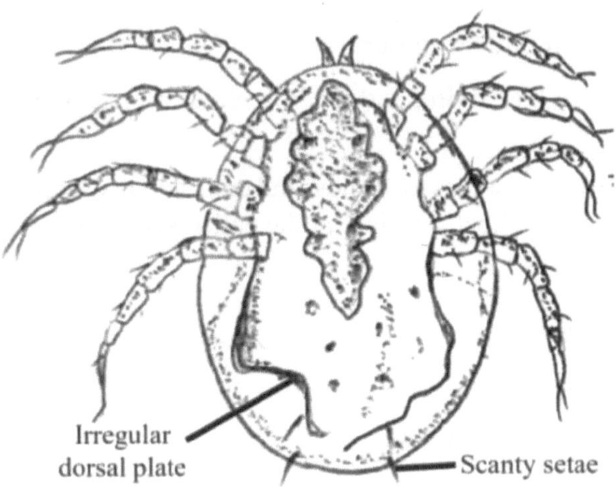

Figure 13.3. *Pneumonyssus caninum*

4. Genus: *Raillietia*

Species: *Raillietia auris*

Host: Cattle

Significance

1. Lives in ears of cattle causing otitis.

Subclass: Acari

Order: Acariformes

Suborder: Actinedida /prostigmata

Characters

1. This suborder is also referred as prostigmata because the stigmata are present at the anterior part of the body.
2. Only few species of this suborder are parasitic.

Family: 1. Trombiculidae

2. Demodicidae

1. Family: Trombiculidae

Characters

1. This family contain mites **whose parasitic larvae are called harvest mites/chigger mite/velvet mites.**
2. They are red, orange or yellow in colour.
3. **Nymphs and adults are free living** and feed on either invertebrates or plants.
4. The larvae mite attaches themselves to the host and their salivary secretion hydrolyses the cuticle of the host forming a tube called **stylostome.**

Genus: ***Trombicula***

Species: *Trombicula autumnalis*

Common name: Harvest mites

Host: Vertebrates including poultry and man

Significance

i. The larvae of this parasite cause generalized pruritis and lesions in interdigital space of the dog and **heel-bug of race horses**.

ii. Transmit *Rickettsia tsutsugamushi* which cause scrub typhus in man.

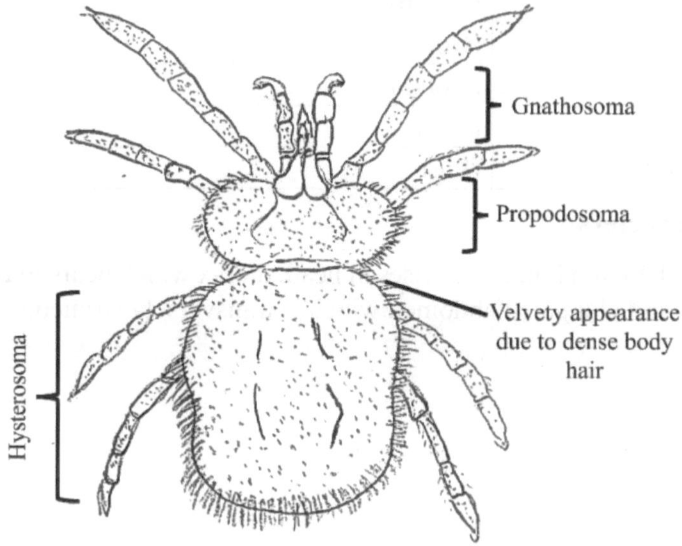

Figure 13.4 *Trombicula*

2. Family: Demodicidae

Genus: *Demodex*

Characters

1. Commonly called **"Follicle mites"** as they live in hair follicles and also in sebaceous glands.
2. They are usually **host specific**.
3. Usually, they are **commensal**.
4. The disease is called demodicosis or demodectic mange or follicular mange. In dog, disease also known as **'red mange'**.

Species

Demodex canis	(Dog)
Demodex cati	(Cat)
Demodex bovis	(Bovines)
Demodex ovis	(Sheep)
Demodex caprae	(Goat)
Demodex equi	(Horse)
Demodex folliculorum	(Man)
Demodex phylloides	(Pig)

Morphological characters

1. Mite is elongated, 0.25 mm long, comprises of head, thorax which bears four pairs of stumpy legs and elongated abdomen which is transversely striated.

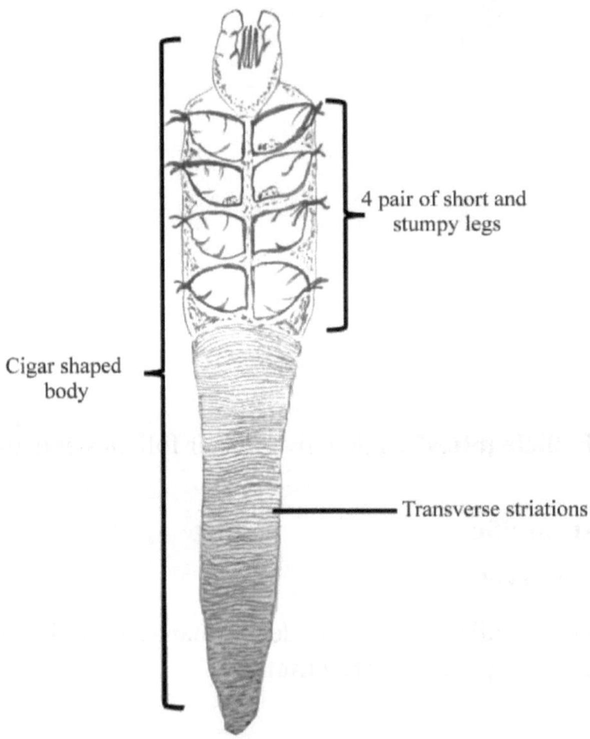

Figure 13.5. *Demodex* (Ventral)

Life cycle: Entire life cycle is spent on the host. Transmission from infected to healthy animal is through direct contact. Life cycle stages include egg, larvae, two nymphal stages; protonymph and deutonymph and adult. Life cycle gets completed in 18-24 days.

Pathogenesis

In Canines

Canine demodicosis usually become evident at the age of **three to nine months**. Pups usually gets infection from the infested bitch where they remain as **commensal.** Severity of lesion is proportional to the number of mites.

Predisposing factors

i. Age, poor condition, intercurrent infection and undue use of alkali soap.

ii. **Cell-mediated immune deficiency.**

iii. Endocrine disease like hyperadrenocorticism and hypothyroidism.

iv. Steroid therapy which is immunosuppressive.

Lesion often start with head and forelimbs and then becomes generalized and spread to entire body. Generalized canine demodicosis is manifested in two forms

a) Squamous form

b) Pustular form

a) Squamous form: This form is characterized by erythema, distension of hair follicles due to mites and cellular debris, hyperkeratosis, hyperpigmentation giving the skin **coppery-red colour**. Animal show alopecia and thickened and wrinkled skin with a **mousy odour.**

b) Pustular form: This form follows the squamous form and is severe phase of the disease. It results from bacterial invasion particularly ***Staphylococcus*** spp. of the dermis. There is infiltration of neutrophills, lymphocytes and plasma cells resulting in pustules formation.

Pruritis is absent in any form of demodicosis. In extensive forms, death results from toxaemia and emaciation.

In Cats: Usually develop lesion like dog, but they are rarely affected.

In Pigs: Large **pustule may occur which are about the size of a walnut** which may later coalesce and rupture.

In Ruminants: Nodules, papules especially on withers, neck, back and flank. Ulceration, fistulae, crusts may be occasionally observed.

In Sheep: Disease is rare and usually scales develop.

In Goat: Pustular form is most common.

In Horses: Asymptomatic, scales develop on face, shoulder, neck and forelimbs.

Diagnosis

i) Clinical signs

ii) **Skin scraping examination**: Before scraping, skin should be squeezed out to push the mites out of the follicles. Lesion then should be scraped gently till the blood oozes out. Examine the scrapings under microscope or boil the scraping material in 10% KOH, centrifuge it and examine the sediment for the presence of mites or eggs. Boiling in 10% KOH is done to dissolve the tissue debris.

Treatment

a) Amitraz® @ 250 ppm for 3-6 treatments

b) Ivermectin @ 0.6 μg/kg b.wt S/C or per os.

c) Closantel @ 5 mg/kg b.wt S/C for 1st injection followed by two dose of 2.5 mg/kg b.wt at weekly interval.

Repeated treatment is required. Broad spectrum antibiotic therapy should also be given to bacterial infection.

Family: Cheyletidae

1. Genus: *Psorergates ovis*

Host: Skin of sheep

Morphological characters:

Body is almost spherical with sides slightly indented between legs. Legs are radially arranged and have paired claws.

Significance: Irritation, biting, scratching, damage to wool and skin.

Diagnosis and treatment: Same as in demodicosis.

2. Genus and species: *Cheyletiella parasitivorax*

Host: Found on fur of rabbits, cats and dogs.

Commonly called 'walking dandruff'

Subclass: Acari

Order: Acariformes

Suborder: Acaridida

Characters

1. Mites of this group lack stigmata hence this suborder also called astigmata.
2. Legs of mites of this suborder bear suckers which are attached with legs through stalks or pedicels.
3. Some species, in unfavourable environment, produce nymphs which are adapted to resist adverse condition. Such nymph is called **hypopial nymph or hypopi** and they are provided with suckers or hooks on their legs which is used to attach to transport host to carry them to favourable situations.

Family

1. Sarcoptidae
2. Psoroptidae

Difference between families Sarcoptidae and Psoroptidae

Sarcoptidae	**Psoroptidae**
These mites usually borrow deep into the skin, so they are burrowing mite.	These mites pass on superficial layer of skin, so they are non-burrowing mite.
Body is globular in shape.	Body is oval shaped.
On dorsal surface, there are grooves, spines and scale i.e. dorsal surface is rough.	These structures are absent so dorsal surface is smooth.
Legs are very short. In *Sarcoptes scabei*, posterior legs (3rd and 4th pairs) do not extend beyond the posterior margin.	Legs are quite big. Posterior leg (3rd and 4th pairs) extends beyond the posterior margin.
Males have bell shaped suckers (caruncles) on 1st, 2nd and 4th pair of leg. On 3rd pair, long bristles are present. In females, bell shaped suckers are present only one anterior i.e. 1st and 2nd pair of legs. On 3rd and 4th pair, long bristles are present.	Presence of bell-shaped suckers on legs is variable as per species.

Sarcoptidae	Psoroptidae
Pedicels are unsegmented.	Pedicels are segmented or unsegmented.
Sexual dimorphism is not pronounced.	Sexual dimorphism is pronounced in male mites, posterior margin is bilobed, 4th pair of leg is smooth than 3rd adanal sheet. Plates are present. In fermale, adanal plates are absent. All legs are equal and posterior margin is not bilobed.
Epimeres are well developed (epimeres are the rod like extension of the coxae).	They are not distinctly seen.
They affect part of skin which is less hairy.	They affect part of skin which is well covered with hair or wool.

Family: Sarcoptidae

Genera

a. ***Sarcoptes***

b. ***Notoedres cati***

c. ***Cnemidocoptes gallinae*** and ***Cnemidocoptes mutans***

Genera

a. *Sarcoptes*

i. Disease caused by this mite is **called scabies in man and sarcoptic mange in animals.**

ii. They are burrowing mite present in deeper layers of skin of animals and man.

Species	Host
Sarcoptes scabei	Man
Sarcoptes canis	Dog and cat
Sarcoptes bovis	Bovines
Sarcoptes ovis	Sheep and goat
Sarcoptes equi	Equine
Sarcoptes suis	Pig
Sarcoptes dromedarii	Camel

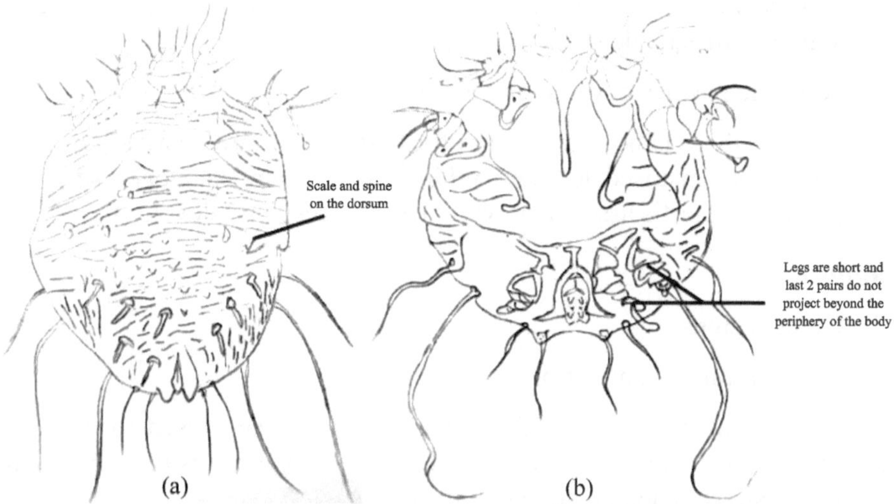

Figure 13.6. *Sarcoptes scabei* (a) Dorsal view (b) Ventral view

Life cycle: The female sarcoptic mites burrow deep into the skin forming tunnels in upper layer of epidermis and eggs are deposited in the tunnels. Around 3 to 5 eggs are deposited per day and likewise 40 to 50 eggs are laid by one female in tunnels. Eggs hatches within 3 to 5 days and larvae come out. A larva has three pair of legs; some of larva come out of tunnel and migrate on surface of skin, but most of them die after some time and majority of them penetrate wall of tunnels and form side pockets or moulting pockets. Inside moulting pockets, larvae moult to nymphal stage. There are two nymphal stages in life cycle namely protonymph and deutonymph. Nymphal stages come out and form new moulting pockets in adjacent areas of tunnel and moult to adult. Female remains inside the moulting pockets, male come out and enter into different moulting pockets and fertilize the female. After fertilization, females start migrating, forming new tunnel or moulting pockets and again process is repeated. This infestation is transmitted through contact. These mites are very susceptible to desiccation and cannot survive for longer period away from host. Entire life cycle is completed in host within 17 to 22 days.

Pathogenesis and clinical signs

1. As the female mites penetrate deep into skin, they suck lymph and also feed on young epidermal cells.
2. They cause irritation and itching forcing the animal to rub its affected part. This cause inflammation of skin which is accompanied by exudate which coagulates and forms crusts on surface.

3. Hyperkeratinization and proliferation of connective tissue as a result skin becomes thick and wrinkled.
4. Alopecia patches develop on the body.
5. Initially there is no pruritis sign for first two or three weeks but as the host gets sensitised to these mites and to their excretory –secretory products, pruritis associated with urticarial response develops.

Diagnosis

1. Clinical signs.
2. Skin scraping examination.
3. Burrow ink test (BIT): This technique is basically used to diagnose scabies in human beings. In this technique, Indian ink is rubbed into the skin lesions to demonstrate the tunnels.
4. Rubbing index: It is used in Australia to diagnose the disease in pigs. Group of pigs are monitored for 15 minutes to record number of rubbing or scratching and is then divided by the number of pigs to obtain rubbing indx. If the index is greater than 0.1 then it indicates need for mange control.
5. Serodiagnosis: ELISA based techniques being used to diagnose the disease.

Treatment

1. Lindane @ 0.01 6-0.08% after every week, 3-4 application is required.
2. Benzyl benzoate @10-20% either in liquid soap or in spirit and applied on affected part of skin.
3. Ivermectin @ 200 μg / kg body weight.
6. Amitraz® @ 3 ml in 1 liter of water, 3 to 4 applications are required weekly interval.
7. Herbal remedies: Neem oil, Karanj oil, AV/EPP/14® (Contains extracts of *Acorus calamus*, *Azadirachta indica, Pongamia glabra*, *Eucalyptus gloulus*).

2. Genus: ***Notoedres***

Species: ***Notoedres cati***

Host: Cat rarely dog and rabbit

Morphology: Similar to *Sarcoptes* except that **there is thumb print like striations on dorsal surface and anus is dorsal and sub-terminal.**

Pathogenesis and clinical signs: same as of *Sarcoptes*

Diagnosis: Skin scraping examination.

Treatment

i. Ivermectin @ 400 µg / kg body weight

ii. Amitraz® @ 3 ml in 1 liter of water, 3 to 4 applications are required weekly interval.

3. Genus: *Cnemidocoptes* (*Knemidocoptes*)

a) Species: *Cnemidocoptes gallinae*

Morphology: Globose body, striations on dorsal side, short and stumpy legs, two longitudinal chitinized transverse bars which runs from the base of pedipalps to the legs. All legs of male possess suckers while female possess none.

Pathogenesis and clinical signs: Causes "**depluming itch**" in the birds. These mites penetrate skin alongside the shaft of the feather. They cause inflammation and exudation so feather from affected area break off or are pulled out by birds therefore, condition is known as Depluming itch.

Diagnosis: 1 to 2 feathers from affected area are pulled out. Base of feather should be scraped in 10% KOH.

Treatment: 1% Sodium fluoride + 10% sulphur + Soap water, equal parts of each should be applied on affected parts of skin.

b) Species: *Cnemidocoptes mutans*

Morphology: Oval body, convex on dorsal side and strongly striated. All legs of male possess suckers while female possess none.

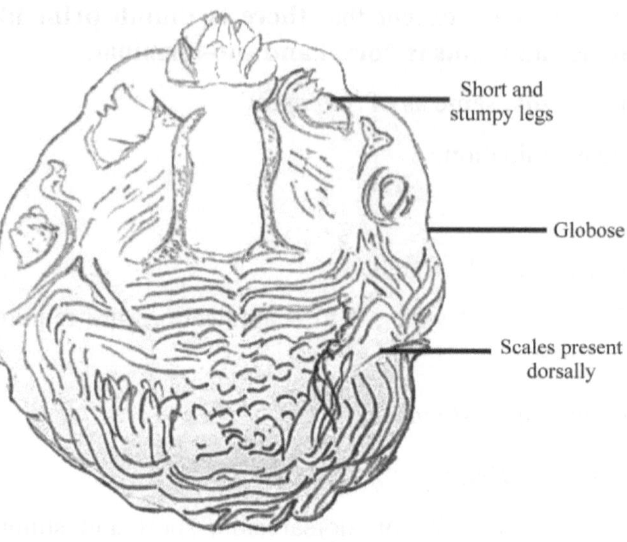

Figure 13.7 *Cnemidocoptes mutans* (dorsal view)

Pathogenesis and clinical signs: Causes **"Scaly leg"** in birds. These mites penetrate into the skin of legs particularly in shank region causing inflammation and exudation of area. As a result, there is hyperkeratinization and scales are formed on affected area of legs.

Treatment: Legs are dipped in 1% lindane in water but before dipping, superficial scales should be removed. 10% sulphur solution is also effective.

2. Family: Psoroptidae

It includes non-burrowing mites and lives in superficial layer of skin causing scab formation.

Note: Characters mentioned in the difference

Genera

a) ***Psoroptes***

b) ***Chorioptes***

c) ***Otodectes***

a) Genus: *Psoroptes*

Species: *Psoroptes ovis* (Host- Mainly sheep, can also affect cattle, horse)

P. cuniculli (Host – Rabbit and Horse)

Characters

1. Mouthpart is pointed.
2. Pedicel long and three segmented.
3. Suckers are present in 1st, 2nd and 3rd pairs of legs in male and 1st, 2nd and 4th pairs of legs in female.
4. Abdominal lobes are rounded.

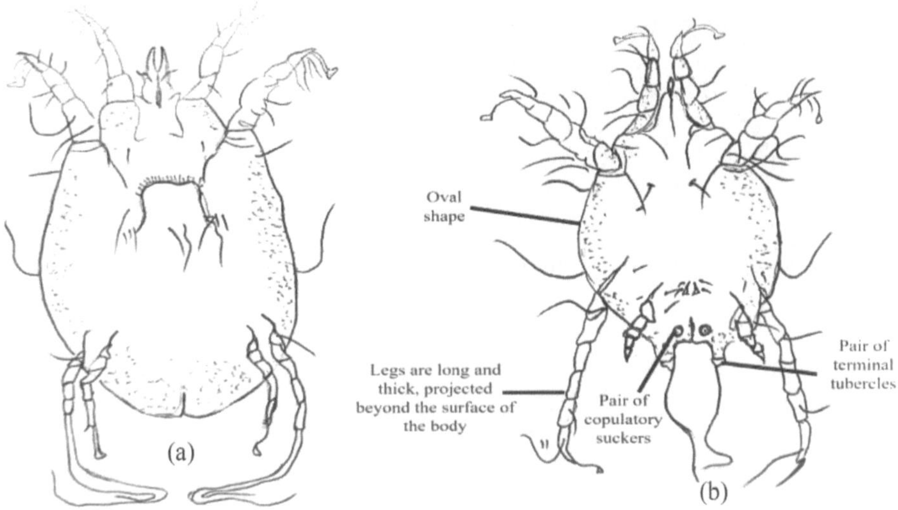

Figure 13.8. *Psoroptes ovis* (a) Dorsal view (b) Ventral View

b) Genus: *Chorioptes*

Species: *Chorioptes bovis* (Host- Cattle, sheep, goat, horse)

Characters

1. Mouthpart is rounded.
2. Pedicel short and unsegmented.
3. Suckers are present on all legs in male and 1st, 2nd and 4th pairs of legs in female.
4. Abdominal lobes are square shaped.

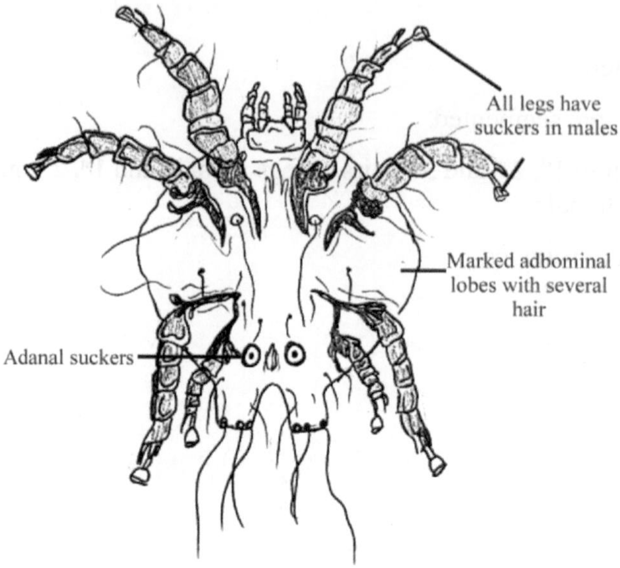

Figure 13.9. *Chorioptes bovis* (ventral)

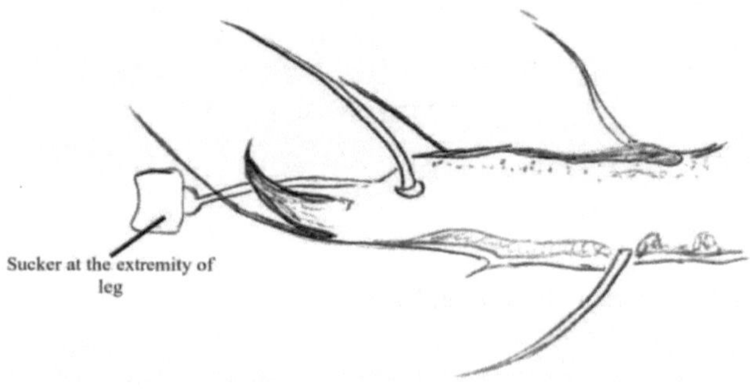

Figure 13.10. Leg of *Chorioptes bovis*

c) Genus: *Otodectes*

Species: *Otodectes cynotis* (Host- Dog and cat)

Characters

1. Mouthpart is rounded.
2. Pedicel short and unsegmented.
3. Suckers are present on all legs in male and 1st and 2nd pairs of legs in female.
4. Abdominal lobes are absent.

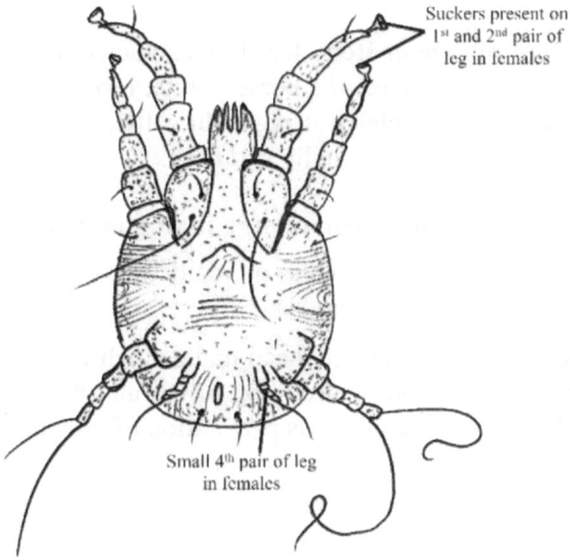

Figure 13.11. *Otodectes cynotis* (ventral)

General life cycle of Psoroptidae: Eggs are laid on the skin. A female lays around 90 eggs during its life time. Eggs hatch in 5-6 days to larval stage which after 2-3 days moults to nymphal stage. Life cycle gets completed in 12 -14 days.

Pathogenesis and clinical signs

a) *Psoroptes* spp.

i. Mite puncture the epidermis to suck lymph and stimulate local inflammatory swelling with infiltration of cells.

ii. Serum exudates on surface, coagulates and form crust or scab so disease in sheep is called **"sheep scab"**.

iii. Marked pruritis, biting, scratching of the lesion and fall out or breakage of wool.

iv. Crusty patches are unsuitable for mites so mites move outward thereby extending the lesion.

v. Debility and emaciation of animals due to restlessness and less feed intake.

b) *Chorioptes bovis*

In horses, this species causes **foot mange or itchy leg**. It is characterized by itching, scab like lesion on fetlock which make the horse to bite, rub, scratch or stamp the legs and kick frequently especially at night. In cattle, lesion is initially found at base of tail then spread to legs, belly and neck.

c) *Otodectes cynotis:* It causes otodectic or ear mange in dog and cat.

i. They attack external auditory meatus, feed on epidermis causing inflammation, waxy exudates which form crusts.

ii. There is intense irritation, animal shakes its head and scratch its ears. This causes haematoma, purulent ootitis, drooping of ear and may be torticollis and epileptic fits. Sometimes there is perforation of tympanic membrane.

Diagnosis

i. Clinical signs.

ii. Skin scraping examination for mite detection.

Treatment: For sheep scab and itchy leg, treatment is same as demodecosis. For, otodectic ootitis, Inj. Ivermectin and local dressing.

14

Pentastomida

Class: Pentastomida

General characters

1. Usually, they are considered as aberrant arthropods as some authors suggest it to be related to annelids.
2. They are elongated, tongue like and transversely striated or sometimes, deeply ringed giving beaded appearance especially at the anterior end.
3. Two pairs of strong hooked claws are present at anterior-ventral surface.
4. Eggs contain fully developed larvae when laid.

Family: Linguatulidae

Genus: *Linguatula*

Species: ***Linguatula serrata*** **(Tongue worm)**

Definitive hosts: Dog, other carnivores and man

Intermediate hosts: Sheep, goat and other herbivorous animals

Location: Upper respiratory tract

Distribution: Worldwide including India

Morphology

i. **Worm is tongue shaped, convex dorsally and flattened ventrally**.
ii. Cuticle is transversally striated.
iii. Male around 2 cm and female 8-13 cm long.
iv. Size of egg around 90 by 70 µm.

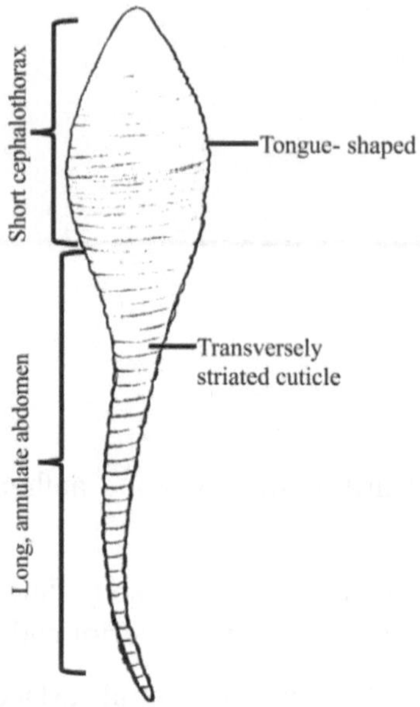

Figure 14.1. *Liguatula serrata*

Life cycle: Eggs are expelled from the respiratory passage of the host and when swallowed by herbivorous animal, hatch in alimentary tract. Larvae then reaches the mesenteric lymph glands in which it develops to infective nymphal stage. Size of larvae is about 500 μm and nymph stage 4-6 mm long. Carnivores gets infected by eating infected viscera of animals.

Pathogenesis and clinical signs

i. Parasites attach themselves to nasal passage.

ii. Light infections go unnoticed but in heavy infections, there is severe irritation, sneezing, coughing, nasal discharge, haemoptysis and dyspnoea. The parasite lives for about 15 months after which the animal usually recovers.

iii. In man, it causes **"halzoun syndrome"** or **nasopharyngeal pentastomosis**.

Diagnosis

i. Clinical signs.

ii. Finding eggs in faeces or nasal discharge.

Treatment

i. Treatment is difficult. Parasite may be removed surgically.

15

Integrated Pest Management (IPM)

Integrated Pest Management (IPM) is an effective and environmentally friendly step towards pest control based on a combination of common practices. IPM programs use up-to-date and comprehensive information about the life cycle of pests and their interactions with the environment. This information, along with existing pest control methods, is used to control pest damage in the most cost-effective manner and with the least possible risk to people, property and the environment. The IPM methods can be used in agricultural and non-agricultural areas, including homes, gardens and workplaces. IPM uses all pest control options, but not limited to the appropriate use of pesticides. In contrast, organic food production shares many of the same concepts as IPM, but limits the use of pesticides to those that come from natural sources rather than synthetic chemicals.

IPM is a set of pest management assessments, choices, and actions rather than a single approach of pest control. Growers using integrated pest management (IPM) that recognize the possibility of insect invasion employ a four-tiered strategy including establishing action levels, keep a look out for and recognize pests, its prevention and control.

IPM establishes an action threshold—a point at which insect populations or environmental circumstances suggest that pest control intervention is necessary—before implementing any pest control measures. It's not always necessary to take action when one pest is seen. Future decisions about pest treatment must take into account the degree to which pests will pose an economic risk. Set thresholds through systematic, regular, and consistent monitoring. Develop thresholds that are appropriate for your circumstance. Modifying thresholds, management and monitoring techniques if necessary. For the majority of pest monitoring techniques, quantitative thresholds can be created, such as treating when specific circumstances are favorable for the onset of a disease or when the number or percentage of invertebrate pests or damaged plant parts surpasses predetermined limits. A good monitoring procedure involves knowledge of pest and beneficial species likely to be present, awareness of the critical crop development stages, good sampling and recording techniques and an estimate of infestation level.

Steps of Pest Control by IPM

1. **Pest prevention before pesticide application**

   - Remove sources of food, water and shelter of pests.
   - Garbage containing food scraps should be placed in tightly covered trash cans. Remove garbage regularly.
   - Fix water lekage and don't let water accumulate anywhere in the home. Don't let water collect in trays. Avoid leaving pet food and water outside for overnight.
   - Clutter provides places for pests to breed and hide and makes it hard to get rid of them.
   - Remove places where pests can enter and hide. For example, cracks and crevices around cabinets or baseboards for ticks and other insects. Use steel wool to fill spaces around pipes. Cover holes with wire mesh.
   - Learn about the lifecycle and habbits of pests to control them.

2. **Safe and correct use of pesticides**

   - Keep pets and children away from areas where pesticides have been applied.
   - After preventive steps have been taken, you can use baits as a first line of chemical defense against insects or rodents.
   - Use the recommended pesticide to kill pests.
   - Use fogging devices for application of pesticide only when necessary.
   - Always read and follow the pesticide label's instructions and safety warnings.
   - Use ready-to-use pesticide i.e., no mixing needed.
   - Only apply chemicals approved for use in animal shelters or agriculture land.

3. **Disposal of left over pesticides and containers properly**

   - Read the label to find out how to dispose of the pesticide and the container.

4. **Avoid pesticides transfer to other containers**

- Store pesticides in original containers only.
- Stricly avoid the empty pesticide containers to store anything else. No matter how well you wash the container, it could still contain remnants of the pesticide and could harm someone.

(A) Chemical control. It is a conventional method of pest control and an important component of the IPM programme. It includes:

(1) Chemical Pesticides. They are used as a last resort in the IPM programme due to negative impact on the environment, health and resistance problem. The different pesticides are:

(a) **Organochlorine compounds**: Organochlorines (OC) are the group of chlorinated compounds widely used as pesticides all over the globe. These chemicals are considered as persistent organic pollutants with high persistence in the environment. DDT, DDD, Dicofol, Eldrin, Dieldrin, Chlorobenziate, Lindane, BHC, Methoxychloro, Aldrin, Chlordane, Heptaclor, Endosufan, Isodrin, Isobenzan, Toxaphene, Chloro propylate are common organochlorines used to kill insects. Though the mechanism of action is not fully understood, organochlorines play a role in facilitating the transport of sodium and potassium ions across neuronal membranes. Organochlorines were earlier used in control of malaria and typhus, yet they are banned in most of the advanced countries. The review statistics on the use of different pesticides shows that 40% of all pesticides used belong to the organochlorine class of chemicals. Due to their low cost and the need against various pests, organochlorine insecticides are among the most widely used pesticides in developing countries of Asia. DDT, BHC, dieldrin, lindane, methoxychlor and toxaphene have high toxicity and thus have been replaced.

(b) **Organophosphates compounds:** Organophosphates include chemicals Dimefox, Mipafox, Methyl Parathion, Ronnel, Enitrothion, Bidrin, Phorate, Fenthion, Caumphos, Abate, Dichlorovas, Diptrex, Phosphomidon, Demetox, Oxydemeton-methyl, Malathion, Dimethoate and Trichlorofan. These compounds are phosphoric acid esters. The OP causes irreversible inactivation of the acteylcholinesterase, and thus inhibit nerve function in insects and many other animals. Now use of organophosphates has been limited due to neurotoxic side effects. Organophosphates are degraded by hydrolysis on the exposure to light, air and soil, however small amounts are detected in food and drinking water.

(c) **Carbamates**: Carbamates are carbamic acid derived organic compounds. Carbamate esters are the functional group used as insecticides. It causes reversible inactivation of the acteylcholinesterase enzyme. Carbamate compounds take weeks or months to degrade in the environment. Examples of carbamate compounds are Carbaryl, Carbanolate, Prupoxur, Dimethan, Dimetilan, Isolan, Carbofuran, Pyrolan, Aminocarb, Aldicarb, Vernolate, Pebulate, Diallate, Monilate, Butylate, Cycloate, Trillate, Thiourea, Methan, Thiram, Ferban, Amoban, Naban, Zineb, Maneb, Ziram Polyran and Dithane M- 45.

(d) **Pyrethroids:** Pyrethroides are organic compounds isolated from the flowers of pyrethrums. The insecticidal properties of pyrethroides are because of ketoalcoholic esters of chrysanthemic and pyrethroic acids. Pyrethroides inhibit the sodium channels and lead to paralysis of the insects. The pyrethroides have a slight level of mammalian toxicity and have a fast biodegradation capacity. Exposure to very high levels of the compounds in air, food or water may cause giddiness, headache, vomiting, muscle twitching, low energy, convulsions and loss of consciousness, The examples are Allethrin, Bonthrin, Dimethrin, Tetramethrin, Ptrethrin, Cyclethrin, Furethrin, Fenevelerate, Alphamethrin, Decamethrin and Cypermethrin.

(e) **Formamidines:** These are insecticides and acaricides that have the characteristic nitrogen structure and are effective against the eggs and larvae of butterflies and moths. They are used as an alternative to organophosphates. They act on the monoaminergic system and activate octopamine receptors leading to functional and behavioral changes in organism. In mammals, the main targets for their toxicity are the alpha$_2$-adrenoceptors which are located pre- and post-synaptically in the CNS and the peripheral nervous system. The examples are Amitraz® and Chlordimeform.

(f) **Macrocyclic lactones:** The macrocyclic lactones are the fermented products of the actinomycete *Streptomyces avermitilis* and *Streptomyces cyanogriseus*. It has an excellent activity against a wide variety of nematodes and arthropods in very low dose rate. Their mode of action still yet to be completely elucidated. However, it acts on γ-aminobutyric acid (GABA) receptor and block interneuronal stimulation of excitatory motor neurons that leads to a **flaccid paralysis**. The macrocyclic lactones enhanced GABA receptor binding results in an increased flow of chloride ions into the cell leading to hyperpolarisation. The examples include Abamectin, Doramectin, Eprinomectin, Selamectin, Ivermectin and Moxidectin.

(2) Herbal pesticides. A number of plants extracts can be used for the control of pests with high efficacy, low toxicity and economic feasibility. Plants like Neem (*Azadirachta indica),* beshram (*Ipomea carnea*), Karanja (*Pongamia glabra*), *Allium sativum* (garlic), *Artemisia absinthium* (Afsantin), *Citrullus colocynthis* (Hanzal), *Laurus nobilis* (Bay leaf) and many more are having insecticidal poperty in their extracts. Neem has multiple mode of actions like oviposition deterrents, repellent, insect growth regulator, antifeedant and poison to larvae and adults.

(3) Botanical pesticides. The alkaloid or terpenoid or phenolic chemical which are produced by the plants to protect themselves against insect attack are called as botanical insecticides. They are widely used against animal pests. These include nicotin (Tobacco plant alkaloid), rotonoid (root of Derris) and pyrethrum (flower of *Chrysanthemum cinerariaefolium*). The mechanism of action of some botanicals are given below:

S. No.	Botanical	Origin	Mechanism of Action	Toxic effect
1	Nicotine	*Nicotiana tabacum*	Acetylcholine mimic; agonist of nicotinic acetylcholine receptor	Contact
2	Azadirachtin	*Azadirachta indica*	Prothoracicotropic hormone (PTTH) inhibitor; phagostimulant disruptor by cholinergic transmission reduction	Insect Growth Regulator/ Repellent
3	Rotenone	*Tephrosia virginiana* *Derris elliptica*	Complex I inhibitor of the mitochondrial respiratory chain	Stomach
4	Pyrethrins I and II	Flowers of *Tanacetum cinerariifolium* roots of *Decalepis hamiltonii*	Voltage-gated Sodium channels modulator	Contact, Stomach
5	Ryanoid	*Ryania angustifolia* *Ryania speciosa*	Activation of sarcoplasmic reticulum calcium channels (ryanodine channels)	Contact, Stomach
6	Sabadilla	*Schoenocaulon calcicola* *Schoenocaulon officinale*	Voltage-gated Sodium channels modulator	Contact, Stomach
7	1, 8 cineole	*Eucalyptus globules* *Umbellularia californica*	AChE inhibitor	Contact, Fumigant
8	Eugenol	*Syzygium aromaticum* *Ocimum basilicum*	Agonist of octopamine receptor	Contact, Fumigant

S. No.	Botanical	Origin	Mechanism of Action	Toxic effect
9	Citronella oil	*Cymbopogon nardus*	Inhibition of (AChE) and glutathione-S-transferase	Contact, Fumigant
10	Thujone	*Artemesia absinthium* *Anamirta cocculus*	Allosteric reversible modulator of GABAA receptors	Contact, Fumigant
11	Terthiophene	*Tagetes minuta*	Light activated phototoxin. Activated species Oxygen generator	Contact
12	Palm kernel crude oil	*Elaeis guineensis* *Elaeis oleifera*	Disturbance of water balance caused by disruption of the protective waxy covering of insects	Contact
13	Ryanodine	Roots and woody stems of *Ryania speciosa*	Voltage-Gated Calcium Channels	Contact Or Stomach
14	Coumaran	*Lantana camara*	Acetylcholinesterase enzyme inhibitor	Contact

(4) Repellent: The repellents are oily volatile substances that require a vehicle for skin application. The most popular synthetic repellents are DEET (N, N-diethyl-meta-toluamide), IR3535 (Ethyl Butylacetylaminopropionate or EB) and Icaridin or Picaridin (1-(1-Methylpropoxycarbonyl)-2-(2-hydroxyethyl) piperidine) and among other products are the natural repellents as lemon, eucalyptus essential oil, citronella and neem. Some chemicals like N-N Diethyl phenyl acetamider (DEPA), dimethyl phthalate. DEET (N, N-diethyl-meta-toluamide) and ethanhexadiol etc.

(5) Insect growth regulators. The chemicals that affect the growth and development of insects are called as insect growth regulators and usually are effective against immature stages. These includes molting hormone, juvenile hormone and chitin synthesis inhibitors. Juvenile hormone and its analog like Methoprene and Fenoxycarb which prevent maturation when added in the breeding medium to increase hormone level in the body. Chitin synthesis inhibitors like Diflubenzuron, Lufenuron, Fluazuron, Buprofezin and Triflumuron, interfere in the chitin production which is an important element of exoskeleton. Other insect growth regulator like Cypromazine which interfere with molting. Pyriproxyfen is a juvenile hormone analogue used for flea control. Thse insect growth regulators cause morphogenetic effects, interfere embryonic development, interfere reproduction, induce egg, larva and pupa diapauses, affect polymorphism and behaviour of insects.

(B) Biological control: It is another control measure by which arthropod population can be reduced. It includes predators, parasitoids, plants, pathogens and genetic manipulation etc. Microbes, bacteria, and viruses have been successfully used to control major medically and veterinary important insects such as ticks, mosquitoes, and tsetse flies etc. A new delivery system, formulations, and the use of genetically manipulated biological control agents, habitat manipulation techniques, and correct timing have contributed to the improvement of business-related biological control products. Mycoinsecticides and mycoacaricides are based on the *Beauveria bassiana* and *Metarhizium* spp., are developed and commercialized to control ticks or insects, like Coleoptera, Hemiptera, Thysanoptera, Lepidoptera, and Orthoptera. The strains of *Bacillus thuringiensis* are found effective to control moths. Different species of parasitoids and predators are also effective against insect pests. Parasitoids and predators also used to control pests in agriculture industry. Parasitic wasps are also used to control insects, such as aphids, moths, and stored grain weevils. The examples of predators, plant base agents, pathogens in medicine and veterinary science are given below:

Predators

- Fish predator like *Gambusiua affins* and *Poecilia reticulte,* guppy fishes for larvae of mosquitoes and *Culicoides.*
- Copepod predators like *Mesocyclops* for larvae of mosquitoes.

Plants: Certain plants are also having larvicidal or repellent action.

- *Melinus, Commiphorea, Pinus,* etc. are having repellent activity against ticks.
- Stylosanthes plants have larvicidal property against ticks like *Boophilus, Rhipicephalus* etc.

Pathogens: Several viruses, bacteria, protozoa and fungi are entomopathogenic and can be used as biocontrol agents.

- **Viruses:** Baculovirus, Reovirus for mosquitoes and black fly control.
- **Bacteria:** *Bacillus thuringiensis* for mosquitoes and black flies.
- **Protozoa:** Ciliates like *Lamborella* and miscrosporidia like *Thelohania* and *Nosema* attack the mosquito larvae
- **Fungi:** *Coelomomyces, Lagenidium* and *Culicinomyces* etc. are mosquito larvicides; *Tolypocldium niveum* is *Oestrus ovis* adulticide and *Metarrhizium anosoplaie* is *Musca domestica* adulticide.

Parasites and Parasitoids

- **Nematodes:** *Hetyertylenchus autumnalis* for *Musca autumnalis* and *Romanomermis* sp. for mosquito larvae.
- **Hymenoptera:** *Musci difurax* spp. for house and stable flies; Ixodiphagus (*Hunterellus*) for ticks.

(C) Genetic control

i. **Resistant breed production:** Production of genetically resistant breed is also tool under IPM. Crossing between *Bos indicus* and *B. taurus* cattle is being practiced to produce tick resistant breed.

ii. **Sterile insect technique:** It is based on the induction of sexual sterility in males through the use of radiation or chemicals and then released into the natural population. Mating with this sterile male do not lead to offsprings.

(D) Cultural management

- Regular and proper disposal of manure.
- Regular shearing of wool at least before the onset of fly season to avoid myiasis.
- Reducing the number of various flies, such as *Culicoides* and mosquitoes, can be achieved by filling potholes, digging burrow pits, ensuring good drainage, periodically emptying water containers, etc.
- Rotational grazing, pasture spelling, burning of pasture and ploughing also help to reduce the pest population.
- Regular grooming.
- Use of insect-proof screens in the shed.
- Use of bits, fogging/misting in barns and and light trap etc. will kill different type of insects.

(E) Immunological control: Although, the vaccines have been developed against few arthropods but the result is encouraging. The mid gut Bm86 antigen vaccine against *Boophilus microplus* (Tickgard®, GAVAC® and Tickgard Plus®) has been shown the efficacy with up to 90%. Another *Lucilia cuprina* larval gut PM44 antigen vaccine has also been developed. Another identified immunological proteins in ticks are Subolesin: a highly conserved protein involved in tick feeding and fertility, Bm95-MSP1A: a tick intestine glycoprotein and *Anaplasma marginale* MSP1A, Ferritin 2: interfere tick iron metabolism, originally identified in *Ixodes ricinus*, VDAC: A mitochondrial protein as a central component of the apoptotic machinery in *R. microplus*.

(F) Manual removal: Removal of ectoparasites like ticks, lice, flea, maggots by simple hand-picking and destroying them by a hard object.

IPM needs to be planned with the long term in mind. The primary objective of Integrated Pest Management (IPM) is to control pests and the environment while maintaining a balance between costs, benefits, public health and the environment. Therefore, the publics awareness and engagement are crucial to the program's success.

16

Acaricide Resistance

Acaricides: Acaricides are agents that kill members of class Arachnida like ticks and mites.

Acaricides are used both in medicine and agriculture, although the desired selective toxicity differs between the two fields.

Different class of acaricides

Class of acaricides	**Chemical Name**	**Mechanism of action**
Organochlorine	Hexachlorocyclohexane, Lindane (BHC), Dieldrin, Aldrin, Bromocyclen, Toxaphene, Methoxychlor,	The organochlorines are thought to act by binding at the picrotoxinin site in the Gamma –aminobutyric acid (GABA) chloride ionophore complex which inhibits Cl^- flux into the nerve. This results in hyperexcitation and ultimately death. **(GABA-gated chloride channel antagonists)**
Organophosphate	Malathion, Coumaphos, Chlorpyriphos, Dichlorovos, Fenthion, Diazinon, Ronnel, Trichlorofon,	Organophosphates and Carbamates acaricides inhibit the acetylcholinesterases enzymes which cause breakdown of acetylcholine and the neurotransmitter continue to cause fire. This results in overstimulation of the nervous systems and ultimately arachnids die. **(Irreversible Acetylcholine esterase inhibitors)**
Carbamates	Carbaryl, Butacarb, Propoxur	
Synthetic pyrethorides	Deltamethrin, Cypermethrin, Permethrin, Fenvalerate	They act on sodium ion channels and thus cause nerve excitation as a result of changes in nerve membrane permeabilities to sodium and potassium ions. **(Sodium channel modulators)**
Avermectins	Ivermectin, Doramectin, Eprinomectin	Macrocyclic lactones stimulate and bind the gamma –aminobutyric acid (GABA) at nerve endings which cause an influx of chloride ions into the cells. This causes hyperpolarisation and subsequent paralysis of neuromuscular systems. **(Chloride channel activator)**
Formamidines	Amitraz	Amidines act by inducing toxic effects on the Octopamine receptor. **(Octopamine agonists)**

Class of acaricides	Chemical Name	Mechanism of action
Phenylpyrazole	Fipronil	It functions by blocking glutamate activated chloride channel. **(GABA blocker)** **Note:** Mammals do not have this type of chloride channel making them much less susceptible to its effect.
Others (Herbal)	Pestoban spray (Contain extract of *Cerdrus deodara, Azadirachta indica, Embelia ribes)* Neem Oil, Karanj Oil, Eucalyptus oil	

What is acaricide resistance?

The ability of a parasite strain to survive and/or to multiply despite the administration and absorption of a drug given in doses equal to or higher than those usually recommended but within the limits of tolerance of the subject.

How does resistance develop?

- Animals are treated with the chemical (Acaricide), exposing nearly all of the tick population to the toxin.
- Susceptible individuals are killed, and those rare individuals that have some genetic resistance, survive.
- They reproduce, and pass along those "resistance genes" to the general tick population.

General Mechanism of resistance

a) **Genetic factors:** Mutation at target site.

b) **Metabolic factors:** Ability of individual to detoxify or sequester an acaricide. The enzyme families known as Cytochrome P450s, Esterases and Glutathione S-transferases are generally involved in metabolic resistance.

c) **Reduced penetration:** Reduced penetration of drug into an individual.

Mechanism of resistance

<table>
<tr><th>Class of acaricides</th><th>Mechanism of resistance</th></tr>
<tr><td>Organochlorine</td><td>Mechanisms of resistance have been suggested primarily due to enhanced metabolism and reduced absorption of chemicals.</td></tr>
<tr><td>Organophosphates</td><td rowspan="2">Target site insensitivity in point mutations in the gene encoding the acetylcholine esterase is suggested to be the reason behind the development of resistance in ticks.</td></tr>
<tr><td>Carbamates</td></tr>
<tr><td>Synthetic pyrethorides</td><td>Mutation in Domain II S 4-5 linker gene and and Domain III of the sodium channel are associated with pyrethroid resistance in R. (Boophilus) microplus. Also, role of P450 cytochrome enzymes in inducing metabolic resistance.</td></tr>
<tr><td>Avermectins</td><td>ATP binding cassette (ABC) transporter efflux pumps has also been reported to have role in Ivermectin resistance in R. (Boophilus) microplus. The transcriptional levels of ABC transporters in the midgut of Ivermectin resistant females was found to be highly up-regulated thus, suggesting its participation in Ivermectin detoxification.</td></tr>
<tr><td>Formamidines</td><td>Studies suggests the involvement of P450s cytochrome monooxygenase along with nucleotide substitutions in octopamine receptor. However, exact mechanism is still not clear.</td></tr>
<tr><td>Phenylpyrazole</td><td>Mutation at target site and involvement of cytochrome P450s enzymes.</td></tr>
</table>

Diagnosis of Acaricide Resistance

A. Bioassays

1) Larval packet test (LPT)

Tick larvae are exposed to chemically impregnated filter papers and their subsequent mortality is quantified after 24 h.

Procedure

- LPT is conducted by impregnated filter paper with different concentrations of test compound.
- Briefly, 0.6 ml of the working solutions (containing test compound) of different concentrations essential oils were used to impregnate 3.75 cm by 8.5 cm filter paper rectangles (Whatman filter paper) and were kept for 30 minutes in the BOD incubator to dry the filter paper.
- Then, the rectangles were folded in half and sealed on the sides with adhesive tapes, forming an open-ended packet for placing the tick larvae.
- Control packets were also prepared by impregnating with the distilled water only.
- 14-day old larvae in 100 numbers (approximately) are dropped into

impregnated filter packets and sealed on the sides using clamps (Stone and Haydook 1962).

- The packets are then incubated at a temperature of 27 ± 2°C and relative humidity of 80 ± 5% and subsequent mortality of larvae are quantified after 24 h.
- The mortality rate was determined according to the following formula:

Mortality (%) = Total no. of dead larvae/No. of total larvae X100

2) Larval immersion test (LIT)

Seven to ten days old tick larvae are immersed in different dilutions of acaricide. Results are evaluated 24 h after each treatment by counting the number of live and dead larvae.

3) Adult immersion test (AIT)

Dose mortality responses of ticks to acaricides are determined by treating engorged female ticks with a range of dilutions of an acaricide. Comparing treated and untreated ticks to assess the effect of a treatment on fecundity and fertility.

Procedure

- AIT is conducted according to the method of Drummond et al. (1976).
- Fully engorged ticks used in the adult immersion test (AIT) within 24 h of collection and incubated until laying eggs.
- A total of 100 adult ticks are weighed and assigned to different groups randomly (10 ticks in each group).
- The collected ticks are dipped for 2 minutes in different concentrations of essential oils (eg. 100mg/ml; 50mg/ml; 25mg/ml; 12.5mg/ml and so on).
- A chemical acaricide and distilled water is taken as positive and negative control, respectively.
- The ticks are allowed to recover from solution and dried by placing on a filter paper in separate petri dishes.
- The ticks that are unable to oviposit 14 days and those that produced non-viable eggs considered as dead.
- LC_{50} value of used compound are determined using probit analysis

by taking concentration in which tick mortality was initiated to the maximum mortality.

- The percentage of mortality was determined by using the following formula: **Mortality (%) = Total no. of dead larvae/No. of total larvae X100.**

B) Molecular Techniques: Allele specific PCR can be used to detect target site mutation. Synthetic pyrethroids resistance can be detected by identification of mutation in sodium channel gene and carboxylesterase genes in ticks. Characterization of a partial segment of the octopamine/tyramine (OCT/Tyr) receptor gene is helpful to identify Amitraz® resistance in *R. microplus*.

C) Biochemical estimation of enzymes: In resistant strains of ticks, level of enzymes gets elevated. Various enzymes like Esterases, Monoamineoxygenase, Glutathione S-transferase, Acetylcholine esterase etc. can be estimated to evaluate the acaricide or insecticide resistance. Beside these other enzymes of Oxidative stress markers can also be evaluated. Superoxide dismutase, Catalase, Reduced glutathione (GSH), Glutathione Peroxidase (GPx) and tissue lipid peroxidation also have value.

Management of Acaricide Resistance in Ticks

1. Judicious use of acaricides

a. Regular monitoring

i. Monitoring the efficacy: Efficacy of treatment of existing acaricide compounds should be regularly monitored so as to delay the development of resistance. Field resistance should be confirmed in lab by using diagnostic assays like larval packet assay, larval immersion test and adult immersion test. These bioassays, though simple and low cost, do not provide information about the genetic basis of resistance. PCR based technique is very sensitive and rapid test that can detect the resistance at an early stage. Allele specific PCR assay (AS-PCR) has been developed to detect resistance causing nucleotide substitution. The most serious limitations of the AS-PCR assay are that it requires detailed knowledge of resistance mechanism at the molecular level. It is better to use bioassays along with molecular tool to detect and allow the quick selection of the best acaricide (Alzoun *et al.*, 2013).

ii. Frequency of treatment: High frequency of acaricide application is a positive risk factor for the emergence of the resistant strains. It has been strongly recommended that acaricide treatments should not exceed more than five per season (Thullner *et al.*,2007).

b. **Rotation of acaricides:** Rotation of acaricides with different mode of action delays the development of resistance due to reduced selection pressure. Most veterinarians suggest that time between changes of acaricides should not be less than two years (Maggi *et al.*,2011). In case of gastrointestinal nematodes, it has been said if a drug, for which the parasite has picked up a resistance, is withdrawn from use for some time, the sensitivity to that drug may return.

c. **Using combinations of acaricides:** Using more than one acaricides with different mode of actions in combinations is another promising approach to delay the emergence of resistance (Lovis *et al.*, 2013). This approach is based on the likelihood that one individual will not have resistant alleles to two chemicals with different mode of actions.

2. Nutritional management

Feeding good quality feed is important for effective immune mechanism. In a field trial in Eastern Queensland (Australia), feeding on poor quality pastures resulted in a significant loss of resistance in the *Bos Taurus* and *B. indicus* x *B. taurus* animals. In another experiment, sheep that was given high protein diet showed resistance to *Rhipicephalus appendiculatus* and *R. evertsi,* maintained weight and did not develop anaemia whereas those maintained on low protein diet suffered tick infestation, lost weight and developed anaemia. T- cell plays major role in mediating acquired resistance to ticks.

3. Herbal acaricides

Due to emergence of drug resistance, drug residue concerns, high cost involved in the development of new drugs and vaccines, emphasis is being laid on the botanicals as herbal acaricide which is generally considered as safe, effective and inexpensive ways of controlling arthropods. Alcoholic extract of several botanicals (*Annona squamosa, Azadirachta indica, Styloxanthes scabra, Acorus calamus, Ricinus communis, Dhatura stramonium, Allium sativum, Carica papaya*) were found to have higher efficacy against ticks. Integration of ethnoveterinary products along with synthetic acaricides may provide beneficial impact in controlling the tick infestations.

4. Genetic resistant breed

Some breeds of cattle carry fewer ticks than others under same environmental management. Such breeds are naturally immune to tick infestation which is manifested more strongly in zebu cattle and their crosses. Resistant cattle, in general, require one or two treatment per season compared with three or four in susceptible breeds.

5. Pasture management

Pasture burning to control ticks is followed in several countries like Australia, South Africa, Zambia and USA. However, in developing countries, burning of pastures on routine basis is difficult for poor livestock farmers. Another approach of the pasture management is pasture rotation which keeps the area free of cattle till the larva die. Pasture rotation combined with acaricide applications was found the most economically feasible IPM strategy in reducing tick burden ranging from 77% to 89%.

6. Vaccine

Vaccine is an important and cost-effective tool against any harmful organisms. Commercial vaccines Gavac® (Heber Biotec; Havana, Cuba), TickGARD® (Hoechst Animal Health; Australia) and TickGARD^{plus} (Intervet; Australia) are based on recombinant form of concealed mid-gut antigen (Bm86) of *R (Boophilus) microplus*. However, these vaccines failed to protect against ticks of different geographic regions. So before introducing these vaccines in new geographical areas, evaluation of vaccine efficacy should be carried out. Advent and use of effective vaccines will reduce the need of acaricides thus delaying the development of resistance and addressing the concern of drug residues.

17

Common Laboratory Techniques in Entomology and Acarology*[1]

1. Collection of arthropods

a. Collection of arthropods from the host's body: The collection of arthropods from the host's body involves various techniques tailored to different species and circumstances. For instance, the extraction of small ectoparasites such as lice, fleas, and wingless keds typically employs usage of forceps with pointed tips for precision. In poultry, a method of brushing against the grain of feathers enables dislodgement of ectoparasites, which are then collected on a black surface for examination. A highly effective strategy for harvesting ectoparasites from small or deceased hosts, such as poultry, involves sealing the carcasses within a polyethylene bag. This confinement prompts ectoparasites to detach from the host and accumulate within the bag, facilitating subsequent collection using a brush. The retrieval of ticks to prevent the rupture of their mouthparts is achieved by straightening the tick forward and pulling backwards before extraction. These ticks are further placed in a tube sealed with a ventilated stopper or a gauze covered with cotton wool plug. The tubes ought to include paper for the ticks to cling onto, along with a labelled piece of paper. These tubes are stored in a cool and humid container for transportation to the laboratory. This container should be well-insulated and equipped with ice blocks or freezer packs as well as damp pads to sustain elevated humidity levels. It's crucial to ensure that the ticks do not directly touch the ice. A sizable thermos flask can be utilized for this purpose. Mange mites, on the other hand, are obtained by conducting deep skin scrapings from the periphery of affected lesions, enabling the collection of specimens for analysis.

b. Collection of free-roaming arthropods: Free-living dipterans, can be captured using fly nets composed of wire mesh attached to a metal ring equipped with a handle or a collection chamber where fine mesh is used as a trap and

*Contributed by Dr. Supriya Sachan, Asst. Prof. and Dr. Kale Chandrakant Dinkar, M.V.Sc. Scholar, Department of Veterinary Parasitology, C.O.V.Sc. & A.H., DUVASU, Mathura (U.P.).

the chamber is protected from direct sun rays and dry air. Alternatively, a petri dish or slide containing serum can also be effective. As flies are attracted to the serum and attempt to feed, their appendages may get trapped, preventing their escape. Another technique involves an aspirator device, comprising a glass tube outfitted with a rubber stopper featuring two apertures. Through these openings, two smaller glass tubes are inserted. One of these tubes is outfitted with a muslin cloth tied at its tip within the collection tube, while the other end of the same tube is affixed with a rubber or plastic tube for oral suction. By positioning the second glass tube near the targeted insect and utilizing oral suction via the rubber tube, the arthropod can be aspirated and placed either over water ice, dry ice or liquid nitrogen or directly put inside the collection tube without causing harm. The specimens should only be preserved through freezing if there is certainty that the pathogen isolation method is compatible with frozen samples.

c. Collection of arthropods from host shelter and surroundings: The oribatid mites typically inhabit the uppermost layer of soil. To collect these mites, soil samples gathered in the morning are spread onto a muslin cloth, which is then positioned on top of the wire gauze of a Baermann apparatus. This apparatus is subsequently placed beneath an electric bulb. The application of heat encourages mites within the soil to migrate, ultimately becoming trapped within the funnel of the Baermann apparatus. Similarly, ectoparasites found in litter and avian nests can be collected using this method. To accommodate larger sample sizes, a drum-like structure may be affixed above the Baermann apparatus, facilitating the collection of ectoparasites.

2. Fixation

Arthropods are immobilized by killing them in a bottle containing cyanide crystals. Typically, cyanide crystals are positioned at the base of a wide-mouthed bottle and covered with dry plaster of Paris. A layer of wet plaster of Paris is then applied above the dry layer and allowed to set. Upon the setting of the wet plaster, 1-2 layers of moist filter paper are added just prior to use. Arthropods are introduced into this bottle, and its opening is tightly sealed with a lid or cork to expose them to cyanide fumes, resulting in their death.

Alternatively, arthropods can be fixed using a solution comprising 30% alcohol and ether (95 ml of 30% alcohol combined with 5 ml of diethyl ether), or by immersing them in hot water at a temperature of 80°C. Another method involves fixation in freshly prepared Bless fluid, consisting of 70% alcohol (90 ml), formaldehyde (7 ml), and glacial acetic acid (3 ml).

3. Preservation

a. **Dry preservation:** After exposing insects like tsetse flies or blowflies to freezing jars or jars containing chloroform, ethyl acetate or carbon tetrachloride wet pads, flies can be secured by pinning them onto pith, a cork-like material, utilizing specialized entomological pins. These pins are inserted through the thorax of the insect and are available in various sizes to accommodate insects of different dimensions. Once pinned, the arthropods are stored in entomological boxes or glass tubes, with naphthalene balls included to deter fungal proliferation. This method of dry preservation aids in maintaining the integrity of setae, spines, and coloration, thereby facilitating better identification. While not entirely reliable for adult mosquitoes, it does assist in preserving the scale and setae patterns essential for identification purposes.

b. **Wet preservation:** Mites, ticks, and ectoparasitic insects are conventionally preserved in ethanol, which is diluted to a concentration of 75% through the addition of water and with incorporation of glycerol at a proportion of one part per ten of the total solution, serves as a valuable adjunct to preclude inadvertent desiccation of specimens. Alternatively, formalin diluted to a range of 2% to 10% in water may be employed, to facilitate its slower evaporation rate compared to ethanol and associated potential hazards. Specimens collected in the field and preserved in formalin can subsequently be transferred to ethanol for laboratory analysis. For temporary preservation, industrial alcohol, medical methylated spirit, or analogous alcoholic solutions are viable options. However, it should be noted that live myiasis larvae may undergo shrinkage if directly subjected to ethanol. To obviate this concern, a solution comprising 90% ethanol and one-part glacial acetic acid can serve as a preservative in fieldwork settings. In laboratory settings, larvae can be killed in water heated to approximately 80°C before transferring them to a solution of 75% ethanol for preservation.

Bijou bottles (5 ml) or universal bottles (25 ml), are preferred due to their resilience to breakage. Plastic containers are deemed suitable solely for field collection purposes, as they may exhibit leakage over protracted storage periods. A provisional label, inscribed in pencil on paper, ought to be enclosed within the tube, delineating particulars such as the collection site, date, and the collector's identity. Post-examination, a permanent label inscribed with waterproof carbon ink (e.g., Chinese or Indian ink) on thin cardboard should be affixed inside the tube, documenting identical collection details. It is advisable to abstain from specifying species nomenclature unless specimens have been definitively identified at the species level. Arthropods have a propensity to coil upon immersion in alcohol, thereby impeding identification efforts. To avoid this obstacle, freshly harvested specimens can be killed in water at approximately 80°C prior to immersion in the preservative solution either in 70% alcohol, a blend of 70% alcohol and glycerine (composed of 90 ml of 70% alcohol combined with 10 ml of glycerol), 5% formalin, or alternatively, in freshly prepared Bless fluid. Saturated solution of chloroform or 10% formalin is used to preserve the colour of ticks.

4. Permanent Mounting of Arthropods

A. For mounting in Berlese fluid, smaller and slender insects such as mosquitoes, which have less body sclerotization, are typically employed. The composition of Berlese fluid includes Gum arabic or acacia (15 gm), Distilled water (20 ml), Glucose solution (10 ml), and Chloral hydrate (10 gm). A drop of Berlese fluid is placed on a glass slide, and the specimen to be mounted is transferred onto it. The legs and wings of the insect are carefully spread using a needle before covering it with a cover glass. Over the course of a few hours, the specimen becomes transparent, and after several days of drying, it can be encircled with nail polish to seal the cover slip. Conversely, in larger insects like flies, various body parts such as antennae, mouthparts, wings, legs and larval posterior spiracles may be dissected and mounted separately in Berlese fluid.

B. After killing, arthropods with highly sclerotized bodies, such as ticks, are immersed in 10% potassium hydroxide (KOH) for either 10 minutes of boiling or an overnight soak. Subsequently, they are transferred to a cavity block and rinsed several times with water to eliminate residual KOH. Then, the specimens are delicately punctured at the posterior end or another suitable location and gently compressed with a blunt tool to expel all internal contents without damaging the body. Following this, they are subjected to dehydration using increasing concentrations of either acetic acid (30%, 50%, 70%, 90%, and absolute) or alcohol (30%, 50%, 70%, 90%, and absolute). Once dehydrated, they can be clarified using carbol xylene or xylene alone before mounting in Canada balsam or DPX.

Alternatively, after dehydration in glacial acetic acid up to 70%, the specimen can be immersed in acid fuchsin for staining, and then dehydrated again using increasing concentrations of acetic acid, clarified in carbol xylene, and mounted.

Examination of specimen: Many arthropods require visual magnification for thorough examination. A basic tool for fieldwork is a hand lens with 10x magnification, which allows for essential identification features to be observed both in the field and later in the laboratory.

For more detailed examinations, a low-power stereoscopic microscope or dissecting microscope is indispensable. These microscopes offer separate light paths and prisms, akin to binoculars, producing a three-dimensional and upright image. They typically feature objective lenses ranging from 0.5x to 5x magnification, paired with eyepieces of 10x magnification. Adequate illumination, ideally through a fibre optic cable to prevent specimen heating, is crucial. These microscopes facilitate examination of specimens in dishes, on slides, or as dry pinned specimens, the latter of which can be easily manipulated by angling the pin in a rubber block.

Specimens preserved in liquid may benefit from surface examination after drying, although prolonged exposure outside the preservative should be avoided. Rinsing in 100% ethanol followed by drying under a lamp or using blotting paper is recommended.

For mites, a compound microscope similar to those used in pathology examination is preferred, with magnifications ranging from 10x to 50x. Phase contrast or ground illumination features are especially useful for mite examination.

Scanning electron microscopes produce highly detailed images of arthropods, but their high cost limits their practical availability for identification purposes, despite their significance in taxonomy.

Collection and Examination of Skin Scrapping for Mites

To collect deeply embedded parasitic mites effectively, a scalpel or knife blade is sterilized by passing it through a flame and then cooled in water. Scraping the edge of the scalpel with a solution of acetic acid and glycerine (1% glacial acetic acid in glycerine) facilitates easier mite collection.

To collect the mites, a fold of skin showing lesions is held between the thumb and forefinger, and the fold's crest is scraped until lymph begins to ooze, being cautious to avoid drawing blood. The scrapings are transferred from the scalpel, using a rotating motion, into a drop of acetic glycerine on a slide. A cover glass is added, along with additional acetic glycerine if needed, and observed under the low power of a compound microscope. For easier diagnosis, scrapings can be boiled with 10% KOH to dissolve debris, and mites can be searched for in the sediment after centrifugation under low power microscopy.

The collected material can be stored indefinitely in acetic-glycerine, with a small crystal of thymol added to discourage fungal growth. Parasites can be separated from debris using a very fine dissecting needle or a finely drawn pipette equipped with a rubber bulb, under a dissecting microscope in good light.

Dissection of Tick's Salivary Gland for Patohological Agents

1. Tick Collection: Use forceps or hands to carefully collect partially engorged ixodid ticks from animals, ensuring not to damage their anterior mouthparts.
2. Preparation: Melt a wax block and place the tick with its ventral surface towards the melted wax.
3. Incision: Make an incision around the lateral margin of the tick, maintaining a 45-degree angle between the blade and the dissection tray. This incision should be superficial.
4. Scutum Removal: Peel off the top scutum of the tick with forceps. The scutum is the dorsal shield-like structure on the tick's back.
5. Locating Salivary Glands: Look for the salivary glands at the anterior lateral margin of the tick under a stereo-microscope. The salivary glands will appear like a bunch of white grapes.
6. Extraction: Carefully remove the salivary glands with the help of fine forceps.
7. Organ Differentiation: Since other organs may come out with the salivary glands, it's important to differentiate them. Other organs include fat bodies, reproductive organs/ovaries, and Malpighian tubules.
    - Fat Bodies: These are white in colour but without any duct.
    - Reproductive Organs/Ovary: They are white in colour with some brown spots with inverted U-shape distal to rectal sac.
    - Malpighian Tubules: These are clear, white tubules.

Staining of Salivary Glands for Microscopic Examination

1. Prepare a microscopic slide by carefully spreading salivary gland tissue using a fine needle to ensure minimal overlapping.
2. Apply a drop of 1% BSA solution to assist in spreading the glands evenly.

3. Allow the tissue to air dry. Submerge the slide in a capping jar filled with Carnoy's fixative for 5 minutes.
4. Rinse the slide in 70% alcohol for 2 minutes, followed by a rinse in distilled water for an additional 2 minutes.
5. Then, immerse the slide in methyl green pyronin staining solution (1ml of 2% aqueous methyl green (0.04%) and 0.5ml of 2% aqueous pyronin (0.02%) mixed with 25ml of 0.1M acetate buffer (pH 4.8) and 25ml of distilled water) for 7 minutes and rinse the slide once more in distilled water for 2 minutes.

   Note: Post slide fixation, Giemsa staining solution, diluted at a ratio of 1:9, can be applied for a maximum duration of 45 minutes, after which it should be rinsed off thoroughly with distilled water.
6. Finally, mount the prepared salivary gland tissue in DPX.

Annexures

Annexure 1: Preparation of Common Laboratory Reagents and Solutions for Arthropods

Solution	Component	Quantity
Bless Fluid	70% Alcohol	90 ml
	Formaldehyde	7 ml
	Glacial Acetic Acid	3 ml
Berlese Fluid	Gum Arabic Or Acacia	15 gm
	Distilled Water	20 ml
	Glucose Solution	10 ml
	Chloral Hydrate	10 gm
Carnoy's Fixative	Absolute Alcohol	60 %
	Chloroform	30 %
	Glacial Acetic Acid	10 %
Methyl Green Pyronin Staining Solution	2% Aqueous Methyl Green (0.04%)	1ml
	2% Aqueous Pyronin (0.02%)	0.5 ml
	0.1M Acetate Buffer (pH 4.8)	25 ml
	Distilled Water	25 ml
0.1M Aceatate Buffer (pH-4.8) in 1000 ml distilled water	0.1 M Acetic acid	5.8 ml
	1.1 M Sodium acetate anhydrous or 0.1 M Sodium acetate trihydrate	8.2 gm or 13.6 gm
Glycerine alcohol	70% ethyl alcohol	90 ml
	Glycerine	10 ml
Giemsa stain	Giemsa stain (powder)	750 mg
	Glycerol	25 ml
	Absolute alcohol	75 ml

Annexure 2: List of Arthropods of Veterinary Importance in Tabular form

S.No.	Scientific Name	Common Name	Host	Disease Transmitted
1.	*Ctenocephalides felis*	Cat flea	Cat, dog, occasionally man, mouse, rat, primates	*Dipylidium caninum*, *Dipetalonema reconditum*
2.	*Ctenocephalides canis*	Dog flea	Dog	*Dipylidium caninum*, *Dipetalonema reconditum*
3.	*Xenopsylla cheopis*	Oriental/black rat flea	Rodents	Bubonic plague (*Yersinia pestis*)
4.	*Ceratophyllus gallinae*	Common flea of chicken	Chicken and occasionally rodents	Endemic or murine exanthematous (*Rickettsia mooseri*)
5.	*Echidnophaga gallinaceae*	Stick tight flea	Chicken, rodent, dog, cat and occasionally rodents	*Francisella tularensis*
6.	*Pulex irritans*	Human flea	Man, pig, dog, cat, rodent	*Dipylidium caninum*
7.	*Tunga penetrans*	Chigger/Chigoe flea	Man, pig	-
8.	*Triatoma*	Kissing bug/cone nose shaped bug/ assassin bug	Man, dog, cat, fox, armadillo, monkey	*Trypanosome cruzi*
9.	*Cimex lectularius*	Common bed bug	Man, and animals	Anthrax, Plague and Typhus
10.	*Menopon gallinae*	Shaft louse of poultry	Poultry and other birds	-
11.	*Menacanthus stramineus*	Body louse of poultry		-
12.	*Heterodoxus spiniger*	Biting louse of dog	Dog	*Dipylidium caninum*
13.	*Lipeurus heterographus*	Head louse of poultry	Poultry and other birds	-
14.	*Lipeurus caponis*	Wing louse of poultry		-
15.	*Gonoides gigas*	Large louse of poultry		-
16.	*Goniocotes gallinae*	Fluff louse of poultry		-
17.	*Columbicola columbae*	Pigeon louse of poultry	Pigeon and other birds	-
18.	*Damalinia (Bovicola) bovis*	Biting louse of cattle	Cattle	-
19.	*Trichodectes canis*	Biting louse of dog	Dog	-
20.	*Haematomyzus elephantis*	Biting louse of African elephants	African elephants	-
21.	*Haematopinus eurysternus*	Short nosed cattle louse	Cattle	-

S.No.	Scientific Name	Common Name	Host	Disease Transmitted
22.	*Haematopinus tuberculatus*	Sucking lice of buffalo	Buffalo	-
23.	*Haematopinus asini*	Sucking lice of equines	Equines	-
24.	*Haematopinus suis*	Sucking lice of pigs	Pigs	-
25.	*Linognathus ovillus*	Face/Blue Louse of Sheep	Sheep	-
26.	*Linognathus vituli*	Long Nosed Cattle Lice	Cattle	-
27.	*Linognathus pedalis*	Foot-louse of Sheep	Sheep	-
28.	*Linognathus. stenopsis*	Sucking louse of Goats	Goats	-
29.	*Linognathus. setosus*	Sucking louse of Dogs	Dogs	-
30.	*Pediculus humanus capitis*	Head Louse	Human	Louse-borne relapsing fever, Epidemic typhus, and Trench fever
31.	*Pediculus humanus corporis*	Body Louse		Louse-borne relapsing fever, Epidemic typhus, and Trench fever
32.	*Phthirus pubis*	Crab/Pubic Louse		
33.	*Culicoides*	Punkies/Biting midges/No-see-ums	Man and animals	*Dipetalonema, Onchocerca cervicalis, O. gibsoni, Mansonella ozzardi*, Queensland itch/ sweet itch/sweat itch/summer dermatitis, Blue tongue, Eastern equine encephalitis, African horse sickness, Bovine ephemeral fever
34.	*Simulium*	Black fly/Buffalo gnat/Turkey gnats	Man, birds and animals	*Leucocytozoon smithi, L. simondi, Onchocerca gutturosa, O. volvulus*, Eastern equine encephalitis and Vesicular stomatitis
35.	*Simulium indicum*	Potu fly	Cattle	
36.	*Phlebotomus*	Sand fly/owl midges	Man, birds and animals	*Leishmania tropica, L. braziliensis, L. donovani*, Yellow fever, *Bartonella bacilliformis* (Carrion's disease/Oroya fever)

S.No.	Scientific Name	Common Name	Host	Disease Transmitted
37.	*Aedes*	Tiger mosquito	Mammals, reptiles and birds	*Plasmodium vivax*, *Plasmodium falciparum*, Japanese encephalitis, Dengue fever, Yellow fever, *Wuchereria bancroftii*, Eastern equine encephalitis, Heartworm, *Setaria*
38.	*Tabanus*	Horse fly/Breeze fly/Gad fly/Cleg	Man, birds and animals	*Trypanosoma*, Equine infectious anaemia, Bovine leucosis virus, Hog cholera virus, *Bacillus anthracis*, *Anaplasma*, Loa loa, *Elaephora schneideri*
39.	*Chrysops dispar*	Deer fly	Deer, man and other animals	*Pasteurella tularensis*
40.	*Chrysops dimidiata*	Mango fly	Man and other animals	*Loa-loa*
41.	*Gasterophilus*	Stomach bot fly of equines	Equines, rarely in dog, pig, birds and man	Gastric myiasis in horses
42.	*Cobboldia elephantis*	Stomach bot fly of Indian elephants	Indian elephants	Stomach myiasis in elephants
43.	*Musca domestica*	House fly	Man, birds and animals	*Vibrio cholera*, *Salmonella typhimurium*, *Bacillus* anthracis, Poliomyelitis, Amoebiasis, Giardiasis, *Habronema megastoma*, *Habronema muscae*, *Raillietina*, *Stephanofilaria*, *Parafilaria bovicola* and *Thelazia* species.
44.	*Musca autumnalis*	Face fly of cattle	Man, birds and animals	
46.	*Morellia*	Sweat fly	Man, cattle and horse	-
47.	*Stomoxys*	Stable fly	Horse	*Trypanososma* *Habronema majus*

S.No.	Scientific Name	Common Name	Host	Disease Transmitted
48.	*Haematobia exigua*	Buffalo fly of India	Buffalo and cattle	*Trypanosoma evansi, Habronema majus*
49.	*Haematobia irritans*	Horn fly	Cattle rarely horses, sheep and dog	*Stephanofilaria stilesi*
50.	*Glossina*	Tse-Tse fly	Man, birds and animals	*Trypanosoma*
51.	*Lucilia*	Green bottle fly	Man, birds and animals	-
52.	*Calliphora*	Blue bottle fly	Man, birds and animals	-
53.	*Callitroga hominivorax*	American screw worm fly	Man, birds and animals	-
54.	*Phormia*	Black bottle fly	Man, birds and animals	-
55.	*Chrysomia*	Screw worm fly	Man, birds and animals	-
56.	*Cordylobia*	Tumbu/Skin maggot fly	Man, rodents, monkeys and dogs	-
57.	*Cordylobia rodhaini*	Lund's fly	Antelopes, rat and man	-
58.	*Booponus intonsus*	Foot maggot	Cattle, goat	-
59.	*Auchmeromyia*	Congo floor maggot	Man and animals	-
60.	*Pollenia rudis*	Cluster fly	Man, birds and animals	-
61.	*Sarcophaga*	Flesh fly	Man, birds and animals	-
62.	*Wolfhartia*	Old world flesh fly	Man, birds and animals	-
63.	*Oestrus ovis*	Sheep nasal bot fly	Sheep and rarely goats	False Gid or pseudo-gid
64.	*Rhinoestrus*	Horse nasal bot fly	Equines	Nasal myiasis
65.	*Cephalopsis titilator*	Camel nasal bot fly	Camel	Nasal myiasis
66.	*Pharyngobolus africanus*	Elephant throat bot fly	Elephant	Nasal myiasis
67.	*Hypoderma lineatum*	Ox warble/Common cattle grub	Cattle, rarely man and horses	Licked beef, Butcher's jelly
68.	*Hypoderma bovis*	Northern cattle grub	Cattle, rarely man and horse	
69.	*H. crossi (Przhevalskiana silenus)*	Goat warble fly	Goat and sheep	Cutaneous myiasis

S.No.	Scientific Name	Common Name	Host	Disease Transmitted
70.	*Hippobosca*	Forest fly/Horse ked	Horse and cattle	*Trypanosoma theileri* and *Haemoproteus*
71.	*Melophagus ovinus*	Sheep ked	Sheep	*Trypanosoma melophagium*
72.	*Pseudolynchia canariensis*	Bird fly/pigeon fly	Pigeon and other birds	*Haemoproteus columbae*
73.	*Dermanyssus gallinae*	Red mite of Poultry	Poultry and other wild birds	*Borrelia anserina*
74.	*Ornithonyssus sylvarium*	Northern mite of Poultry	Poultry and other birds	Fowl pox virus and Western equine encephalomyelitis
75.	*Otobius megnini*	Spinose ear tick	Dog, sheep, horse, cattle, sometimes goat, pig, cat man and other wild animals	Otitis
76.	*Ornithodorous moubata*	Eyless tampon	Animals and man	*Aegyptinella pullorum*, *Borrelia anserina*, Anaplasmosis, reservoir host of African swine fever virus vector of *Borrelia duttoni* (causes relapsing fever in human) and Q fever.
77.	*Ixodes ricinus*	Castor bean tick	Dog, domestic and wild animals	*B. divergens*, *B. bovis*, *Anaplasma marginale*, Louping ill virus, Tick-borne fever, Tick pyaemia
78.	*Ixodes hexagonus*	Hedgehog tick	Dog, Man	Lyme disease and tick-borne encephalitis (TBE) in man
79.	*Ixodes canisuga*	British dog tick	Dog	-
80.	*Ixodes pilosus*	Bush tick	Cattle, sheep, horse, dog, cat and wild ungulates	-
81.	*Ixodes scapularis*	Shoulder/Black-legged tick	Cattle, sheep, horse, dog, cat	Lyme disease
82.	*Boophilus annulatus*	North American tick	Domestic and wild ungulates	*Babesia bigemina*, *Borrelia theileri* and *Anaplasma*

S.No.	Scientific Name	Common Name	Host	Disease Transmitted
83.	*Boophilus decoloratus*	Blue tick	Cattle, equine, sometimes, sheep, goat and wild ungulates	*Babesia bigemina*, *B. ovis*, *Anaplasma marginale*, *Borrelia theileri* and *Babesia trautmanii*
84.	*Boophilus microplus*	Tropical cattle tick	Cattle, horse, goat, sheep and deer	*Babesia bigemina*, *Borrelia theileri* and *Anaplasma*
85.	*Rhipicephalus appendiculatus*	Brown ear tick	Cattle, dog, equine, sheep, goat and wild animals	*Theileria parva*, *T. taurotragi*, *T. mutans*, *B. bigemina*, *Anaplasma bovis* (*Ehrlichia bovis*), *Hepatozoon canis*, Exanthematic fever in dog, *Rickettsia conorii*, virus of Nairobi sheep disease and Louping ill in sheep
86.	*Rhipicephalus sanguineus*	Brown dog tick	Mammals and birds	*Ehrlichia canis*, *Babesia canis*, *Babesia gibsoni*, *Hepatozoon canis* and *Rickettsia conorii*
87.	*Rhipicephalus evertsi*	Red-legged tick	Domestic and wild animals	*Babesia caballi*, *B equi*, *Theileria equi*, *T separate*, and *T. parva* (secondary vector) *Anaplasma marginale*, *Borrelia theileri*, *Rickettsia conorii*, and Kerai, Wad Medani, and Thogoto viruses.
88.	*Haemaphysalis leachi*	Yellow dog tick	Domestic and wild carnivores, small rodents and rarely cattle	*Babesia canis*, *Rickettsia conorii* and *Coxiella brunetii*
89.	*H. longicornis*	Bush tick or New Zealand tick	Man cattle, sheep, goat and birds	*Theileria* and *Coxiella brunetii*
90.	*Haemaphysalis punctata*	Red sheep tick	Sheep, goat, deer cattle	*Babesia motasi*, *Theileria ovis*, *Theileria buffeli* and *Anaplasma*

S.No.	Scientific Name	Common Name	Host	Disease Transmitted
91.	*H. leporis-palustri*	Rabbit tick	Rabbit	*Coxiella brunetii,* Rocky Mountain spotted fever and Tularemia
92.	*Dermacentor andersoni*	Rocky mountain wood tick	Small mammals, horse, cattle	*Anaplasma*, *Babesia canis*, *Leptospira pomona* and *Coxiella brunetii*
93.	*Dermacentor variabilis*	American dog tick	Dogs, wild rodents	Rocky Mountain Spotted Fever (*Rickettsia rickettsii*), *Francisella tularensis*, *Ehrlichia canis*.
94.	*Dermacentor occidentalis*	Pacific coast tick	Deer, cattle, horse, donkey, rabbit, sheep, man	*Anaplasma*, Colorado tick fever, Q fever and Tularaemia
95.	*Dermacentor nigrolineatus*	Brown winter tick	Horse, cattle	-
96.	*Amblyomma hebraeum*	Bont tick	Domestic and wild mammals, birds	*E. ruminantium*, *Theileria mutans*, *Rickettsia conorii* and *Rickettsia africae*
97.	*Amblyomma variegatum*	Variegated/ tropical bont tick	Mammals and rarely birds	*Ehrlichia ruminantium* (= *Cowdria ruminantium*), *Ehrlichia bovis*, *Theileria mutans*, *Theileria velifera* and *Coxiella brunetii*
98.	*Amblyomma americanum*	Lone star tick	Fox and other mammals	Q fever, Rocky Mountain spotted fever and Tularemia fever
99.	*Amblyomma maculatum*	Gulf coast tick	Birds, rodents, cattle, horse, sheep, dog, man	Tick paralysis
100.	*Amblyomma cajennense*	Cayenne tick	Fox and other mammals	*Leptospira pomona*
101.	*Trombicula*	Harvest/chigger mites/aoutat/ lepte automnale/ bug of race horses	Man, domestic animals, birds	*Rickettsia tsutsugamushi*
102.	*Pediculoides ventricosus*	Grain itch mite	Man and domestic animals	Intense pruritis
103.	*Demodex*	Cigar shaped mite	Mammals	Red mange

S.No.	Scientific Name	Common Name	Host	Disease Transmitted
104.	*Cheyletiella yasguri*	Walking dandruff of dog	Dog	Mild dermatitis and extensive popular eruptions
105.	*Cheyletiella blakei*	Walking dandruff of cat	Cat	
106.	*Sarcoptes*	Burrowing mite	Domestic and wild mammals	Scabies in man and sarcoptic mange in animals
107.	*Cnemidocoptes gallinae*	Depluming itch	Poultry	Depluming itch
108.	*Cnemidocoptes mutans*	Scaly leg	Poultry	Scaly leg
109.	*Cytodites nudus*	Air sac mite	Poultry	Pulmonary disorders
110.	*Laminosioptes cysticola*	Subcutaneous mite	Poultry	Nodules
111.	*Liguatula serrata*	Tongue worm	Dog, other carnivores and man	Halzoun syndrome or nasopharyngeal pentastomosis

Annexure 3: Important Vector-Borne Diseases of Canine

Disease	**Pathogen**	**Vector**	**Zoonotic potential**
Granulocytic anaplasmosis	*Anaplasma phagocytophilum*	Ticks	Zoonotic
Ehrlichiosis	*Ehrlichia canis*	Ticks	Zoonotic
Thrombocytic anaplasmosis	*Anaplasma platys*	Ticks	Zoonotic
Rickettsiosis	*Rickettsia rickettsii*	Ticks	Zoonotic
Tick-borne encephalitis	Flavivirus	Ticks	Zoonotic
Looping ill	Flavivirus	Ticks	Zoonotic
Canine babesiosis	*Babesia canis*, *Babesia vogeli, Babesia rossi, Babesia gibsoni*	Ticks	Not reported
Canine Hepatozoonosis	*Hepatozoon canis, H. americanum*	Ticks	Not reported
Canine Bartonellosis	*Bartonella henselae, Bartonella clarridgeiae*	Ticks and fleas	Zoonotic
Canine Rickettsiosis	*Rickettsia* typhi, *Rickettsia felis*	Flea (*Ctenocephalides felis*)	Zoonotic
Tapeworm infection	*Dipylidium caninum*	Flea and Lice	Zoonotic
Canine Heartworm disease	*Dirofilaria immitis, Dirofilaria repens*	Mosquitoes (*Culex* spp., *Aedes* spp. and *Anopheles* spp.)	Zoonotic
Leishmaniosis	*Leishmania tropica, L. donoveni*	Sand fly (*Phlebotomous* sp.)	Zoonotic
Trypanosomiasis	*Trypanosoma evansi*	Biting flies (*Tabanus, Stomoxys*)	Not reported
Canine Oriental eye worm	*Thelazia callipaeda*	House fly (*Musca autumnalis* and *Musca hervei*)	Zoonotic
Chagas disease	*Trypanosoma cruzi*	Reduvid bug	Zoonotic

Annexure 4: Important Vector-Borne Diseases of Cattle

Disease	**Pathogen**	**Vector**
Bluetongue disease	Bluetongue virus	Culicoides
Bovine Besnoitiosis	*Besnoitia besnoiti*	Tabanids and other blood sucking flies
Bovine theileriosis	*Theileria parva* and *T. annulata*	Ticks (*Rhipicephalus* and *Hyalomma*)
Bovine thelaziosis	*Thelazia* sp.	*Musca* sp.
Bovine parafilariosis	*Parafilaria bovicola*	*Musca* sp.
Pink eye	*Moraxella bovis*	*Musca* sp.
Anaplasmosis	*Anaplasma marginale* and *A. centrale*	Variety of tick species
Bovine babesiosis	*Babesia bovis, B. bigemina*	Ticks (*Rhipicephalus* sp.)
Bovine trypanosomosis	*Trypanosoma evensi*	Biting flies (*Tabanus, Stomoxys*)

Index

A

Acari 92, 129, 132, 137
Acaricide Resistance 159, 160, 161, 163
Acaricides 97, 99, 127, 152, 159, 160, 161, 162, 163, 164, 165
Acarology 2, 167
Acetylcholinesterase enzyme inhibitor 154
Adult immersion test (AIT) 162
Aedeagus 4, 65
Aedes 6, 14, 22, 23, 27, 178, 184
Aegypinella pullorum 97
African Horse Sickness 17
Allele specific PCR 163
Allergic Dermatitis 17
Alopecia 135, 140
Alphamethrin 152
Amblycera 74
Amblyomma 94, 105, 119, 120, 121, 122, 125, 128, 182
*Ametamorphos*is 12
Aminocarb 152
Amitraz 127, 136, 140, 141, 152, 160, 163
Anaemia 1, 32, 60, 61, 70, 71, 82, 97, 126, 164, 178
Anal Groove 100, 105, 107, 108, 110, 113, 115, 117, 120
Anal Shield 105
Anal Struts 169
Anapalsma 97
Anaplasma 32, 100, 106, 109, 111, 112, 119, 123, 124, 125, 157, 178, 180, 181, 182, 184, 185
Animalia 92
*An*nulations 28, 29
Anopheles 6, 14, 22, 23, 24, 25, 27, 184
Anoplura 73, 79
Antifeedant 153
Antihistaminic Agents 127
Apodous Larva 12
Aponomma 122, 125
Apterygota 13
Argas 94, 95, 96, 97, 99, 100, 126
Argen*tine T*ick 113
Arthropoda 2, 5, 7, 92
Assassin Bug 86, 176, 177
Astigmata 137
ATP binding cassette (ABC) 161
Autolysis 43
Azadirachtin 153

B

B. annulatus 111
Babesia 6, 109, 110, 111, 112, 114, 116, 118, 119, 123, 124, 125, 180, 181, 182, 184, 185
Bacillus 32, 36, 128, 155, 178
Baculovirus 155
Baermann Apparatus 168
Basis Capituli 93, 100, 101, 105, 107, 110, 111, 113, 115, 117, 119, 123, 124
Bed Bugs 12, 85
Beetles 6, 12, 13, 63
Berlese Fluid 170
BHC 151, 159
Biochemical estimation of enzymes 163
Biological Control 27, 128, 155
Black Flies 21, 155
Blue Bottle Fly 40, 179
Blue Louse of Sheep 80, 177
Blue Tick 112, 180
Body Louse of Poultry 74, 176, 177
Body Louse of Sheep 80
Boophilus 6, 94, 103, 105, 110, 111, 112, 123, 128, 155, 156, 161, 165, 180, 181
Botanical Pesticides 153
Bot Fly 47, 57, 178, 179
Bovine Ephemeral Fever 17, 177
Bovine leucosis virus 32, 178
Brachycera 14, 28
Breech Strike 45
Breeze Fly 178
Brown Dog Tick 110, 124, 181
Brown Ear Tick 108, 181
Brown Winter Tick 119, 182

Buffalo Fly 178
Bugs 6, 12, 13, 85
Burrowing Mite 137, 138, 183
Burrow Ink Test (BIT) 140
Butcher's Jelly 52, 179

C
Calliphorinae 40
Canada Balsam or DPX 170
Canine Demodicosis 135
Carbamic Acid 152
Carbaryl 152, 159
Carbofuran 152
Carbol Xylene 170
Carbon Bisulphide 56
Carbon Tetrachloride 169
Carboxylesterase genes 163
Carnoy's Fixative 173
Castor Bean Tick 106, 123, 180
Caumphos 151
Ceratopogonidae 14, 15
Chemical Control 151
Chilopoda 6
Chitin Synthesis Inhibitors 154
Chlorobenziate 151
Chloroform 36, 45, 169, 170
Chlorolane 71
Chloro propylate 151
Ch*orioptes* 142, 143, 144, 146
Chrysanthemum 153
Chrysops 14, 28, 29, 178
Cimex lectularius 85, 86, 176, 177
*C*lass Insecta 7, 12, 13
Clegs 28, 29
Cn*emidocoptes (*Kn*emidocoptes)* 141
Cobboldia elephantis 57, 178
Cochliomyia (Callitroga) hominivorax 40
Comb 65, 66, 70
Culicinae 22, 26
Cutaneous Myiasis 42, 45, 57, 179
Cytochrome P450s 160, 161

D
Damalina *78*
Deer Flies 28
Dem*odex* 133, 134, 182
Depluming Itch 141, 183
Dermacentor 94, 105, 117, 118, 122, 124, 125, 126, 182
Dermanyssus 129, 130, 180
Dimethrin 152
Dipetalonema 17, 70, 176, 177

E
Ecdysis 2, 5
Echidnophaga 66, 67, 69, 70, 176, 177
Elephant Bot Fly 57
Entomology 1, 2, 6, 167
Esterases 160
Exoskeleton 2, 5, 12, 154
Eyeless Tampan of Africa 99

F
Foot Louse of Sheep 81
Foot Mange 146

G
GAB*A Blocker* 160
*Gama*sid Mite 129
Gasterophilus 14, 53, 54, 57, 178
Gastric Myiasis 53, 57, 178
Gen^e^tic Control 27, 128, 156
Glutathione (GSH) 163
Grasshoppers 89

H
Haemato*pota* 14, 28, 29
Haemocoel 3, 4
Haller's organ 93
Halters or Balancers 13
Halzoun Syndrome 148, 183
Hard Ticks 94, 101, 123
Head Louse of Poultry 76, 176, 177
Heart Worm 27, 178
Heel-bug of race horses 133
Hemelytra 85
Heterodoxus 75, 176
Holomenopon 75
Horn Fly 179
Hyalomma 94, 104, 109, 113 114, 123, 127, 185
Hyperkeratosis 135
Hypoder*ma* 47, 50, 51, 52, 53, 57, 179

I
Insecta 2, 5, 6, 7, 11, 12, 13, 63, 73, 85, 92
Insect Development Inhibitor (IDI) 71
Insect Growth Regulator 153, 154

Ixodes 94, 104, 105, 106, 123, 126, 157, 180

J
Jigger/ Chigoe 66

L
Larval immersion test (LIT) 162
Larval packet test (LPT) 161
Larviparous Insects 11
Licked Beef 52, 179
Linguatula *6, 147*
Lone Star Tick 121, 182
Lucilia 40, 41, 43, 57, 156, 179

M
Maggot Wound 36
Moulting in Arthropods 5
Musca 9, 12, 33, 34, 35, 40, 43, 57, 155, 178, 184, 185
Myia*sis* 1, 2, 32, 39, 42, 43, 44, 45, 46, 47, 53, 57, 82, 156, 169, 178, 179

N
Notoedres ca*ti* 138, 140

O
Obligatory Ecto-Parasites 73
Obtectate Pupa 12
Octopamine/tyramine (OCT/Tyr) receptor gene 163
Oestrus 11, 47, 48, 49, 57, 155, 179
Old World Flesh Fly 179
Old World Screw Worm Fly 40
One Host Tick 103, 111, 112, 119, 123, 125, 127
Ornithodoros 94, 95, 99, 100, 126
Otobius 94, 95, 97, 98, 99, 100, 180

P
Phlebotomus 14, 18, 19, 177
Pho*rmia* 40, 43, 179
Pizzle Strike 45
Pneumonyssus 131, 132
Polypodous Larva 12
Prothoracicotropic Hormone (PTTH) Inhibitor 153
Pseudolynchia 14, 60, 180

Q
Queens Land Itch 17

R
Reduvid Bug 86, 184
Repellent 18, 153, 154, 155

S
Sarcophaga 43, 46, 57, 179
Sarcoptidae 137, 138
Scabies 138, 140, 183
Scaly Leg 142, 183
Screw Worm Myiasis 32, 42
Stomoxys 9, 12, 33, 34, 35, 36, 38, 178, 184,
Strike 42, 45

T
Tabanus 9, 14, 28, 29, 30, 31, 32, 184, 185
Tunga 66, 69, 176
Two Host Tick 103, 104, 109, 124

V
*V*omit Drop 103, 104, 109, 124

W
Warbles 51, 52, 53
Winter Resting Sites 51

X
Xenopsylla 66, 68, 70

Y
Yellow Dog Tick 116, 124, 181
Yellow Fever 6, 27, 177, 178